Praise for Ope

"Dr. Taher's remarkable journey fro
conquering Mount Kilimanjaro is an in
book he shares everything you need to conquer your own challenges."

—Neal D. Barnard, MD, FACC,
Adjunct Professor of Medicine, George Washington University
School of Medicine, and *New York Times* best-selling author

"This is an insightful recount of a journey on a road to recovery that needs
to be traveled for many more of us. Pay particular attention to the chapter
titled 'Diet is More Important Than Exercise.' We really can't exercise
our way out of a bad diet. The two should complement each other, and
always seek the latest evidence in this evolving area, as one by one, all
diets—other than the whole-food, plant-based diet—end up with risks
that are avoidable."

—Kim Allan Williams Sr., MD, MACC, FAHA, MASNC, FESC,
James B. Herrick Professor of Heart Research, Chief, Division
of Cardiology, Rush University Medical Center

"Imagine a very senior, dedicated family doctor, late in his career,
unexpectedly suffering a serious heart disease that requires heart surgery.
Now imagine how he faces it, as a longtime medical professional, in a
manner that is self-reflective, courageous, and inspirational. In doing so,
he reverses his illness by traveling a pathway paved by Nature herself.
Finally, imagine having a family doctor like Akil Taher. His book,
Open Heart, *is an inspirational quick read with a message that will*
be remembered."

—T. Colin Campbell, PhD, Jacob Gould Schurman Professor
Emeritus of Nutritional Biochemistry, Cornell University,
and coauthor of the best-selling book *The China Study*

"A personal account of a physician writing with brutal honesty and a genuine urge to help multitudes of needy people. It leads by demonstrating how a person, especially a physician, can lift himself from the nadir of negativism to a zenith of zeal, to blissfully enjoy a self-created renewed life. The author will hold your hand compassionately while you trace that journey."

—Bhagirath Majmudar, MD,
Emeritus Professor of Pathology and Gynecology-
Obstetrics, Emory University, and a priest and a poet

"Heart disease is the leading killer in the United States and India, and truly avoidable. Bypass surgery implies cutting open the sternum and reaching into the thorax. When humans play God, there is always a risk. Dr. Taher went through it all and found out that there is a better way to live where we can all thrive. Lifestyle changes that not only brought him joy, but saved his life."

—Dr. Nandita Shah,
recipient of the prestigious *Nari Shakti Award* 2016,
India's highest civilian honor for women, and author
of the book *Reversing Diabetes in 21 Days*

"Dr. Taher has written a thoughtful, readable, information-rich account of his amazing journey from heart disease patient to marathon runner and mountain climber. This book is inspirational. If you are contemplating lifestyle changes that include adopting a whole-food plant-based diet, challenging physical activity, and emotional wellbeing, start by reading this book."

—Jennifer Rooke, MD, MPH, FACOEM, FACPM,
Assistant Professor of Community Health and Preventive
Medicine, Morehouse School of Medicine

"An excellent blending of personal challenge from a heart patient, adventure from a marathoner and mountain climber, and good medical and diet advice from a physician."

—Beheruz N. Sethna,
President Emeritus and Regents' Professor of
Business, the University of West Georgia

"This beautifully written book is a physician's message to anyone who wishes to find health, adventure, and joy after looking disease and death in the eye. Instead of an easy fix, it offers a serious guide to shifting one's life gears after the age of sixty."

—Arjun Appadurai,
Paulette Goddard Professor of Media, Culture, and
Communication, New York University

"Dr. Taher's book opens not just a view of what one's choices in life should be, he truly opens his own life to the reader. The honest description of his earlier life sheds the professional elitism so common in society. He describes his transformation and the changed person he became with scientific clarity. I could not put the book down. Highly recommended."

—Winston Tellis, PhD,
Professor Emeritus of Information Systems and
Operations Management, Fairfield University

"Dr. Taher reveals his own true story, about a health crisis that turned his life around and led to a remarkable journey of self-discovery. A truly inspiring story that we should all read."

—Aasif Mandvi,
actor, comedian, and writer

OPEN HEART

The Transformational Journey of a Doctor
Who, After Bypass Surgery at 61, Ran
Marathons and Climbed Mountains

AKIL TAHER, MD

To my wife, Nafisa, for believing in my dreams and standing by me every step of the way. Your warm spirit and loving encouragement have uplifted me at the toughest of times.

To Akil Taher (1948-2009), I owe a greater debt than I can express. A sincere and hardworking physician who realized at age sixty-one that he needed to make major changes in his life. That burnt-out individual, afflicted with myriad health issues and specific vulnerabilities, helped me become the man, the husband, the father, the grandfather, and the friend that I am today, and to that Akil, I express a special nod of gratitude. He is the sole reason this book has come to life, transforming me into an author.

So, I dedicate this book to my earlier self, who overcame hurdles on his path so he could live a healthy, energetic, and fulfilling life, and who cried and laughed in equal measure as he strove to create the new Akil ... me.

Adventure may hurt you, but monotony will kill you.

– Akil Taher, MD

Contents

INTRODUCTION

I wasn't medically *unaware* that heart disease is the leading cause of death in the United States, India, and many other countries. I wasn't obese or a chain smoker. I didn't lack the resources to get the best *personal* health care, and I didn't unduly worry or care about a dietary and fitness regime, despite having high cholesterol. I was a know-it-all physician who believed that medical science had advanced greatly and had the necessary solutions for chronic diseases, including heart disease.

Like most people, my belief that *heart disease won't happen to me* compounded matters, until it came calling at the ages of fifty-six (leading to stents angioplasty) and sixty-one (culminating in open-heart surgery in 2009). I felt that my whole world had turned upside down. After the surgery, I realized I had two choices—first, lead a cautious, mediocre, and sedentary life, as I'd seen in most patients after a heart-bypass surgery; or second, change my lifestyle to incorporate healthy eating habits, an exercise regimen, meditation, and regular practice of yoga.

I could have retired immediately, sat on my rocking chair all day, lived vicariously through my children and grandchild, and resigned myself to the inevitability of eventual death. Instead, I chose to live life to the fullest, turning a setback into an opportunity. Opting for the second choice, I embraced life with an infectious, positive mindset, even as I continued in my role as a physician.

Over the next decade, my heart problem became the most important motivator for transforming my life. My journey—the recovered bypass-surgery patient scaling mountain peaks, running marathons, participating in a triathlon, and becoming a century bike rider—led me to explore unknown paths and discover myself, experiment with various types of diets and exercises, helped me better understand medical science and alternative medicine, aided me in staying open to learning, and propelled me to write this book, to share the story of a resurgent physician, a septuagenarian athlete, and a holistic health and wellness consumer.

As I confronted and dealt with various health issues, I grew in courage, determination, and tenacity, as well as in empathy and compassion. I let go of the need to control, tried to see the positive in each scenario, and stopped overanalyzing every situation I encountered. I also developed a clear understanding of things that actually mattered, and I realized that it was possible to have clarity despite the hurdles that came my way, real and imagined.

This book is an invitation for you to come take this journey with me, to experience the agony of living in an exhausted body with a long list of seemingly insurmountable problems, and learn how I overcame these challenges with the adoption and espousal of an *integrated* healthy life—physical health, spiritual health, emotional health—so that you can avoid the big mistakes I made and instead, make the small yet important changes to protect your heart and improve your overall health and well-being.

This book also provides science-based reasons, backed by personal experiences, for eating a whole-food, plant-based (WFPB) diet, which is a significant contributor toward living a *healthy* long life. I have delved into the importance of meditation, too, as a method to sustain mental and emotional nourishment in the furtherance of my spiritual well-being.

Chronic diseases such as cancer, diabetes, arthritis, kidney disease, heart disease, and stroke are what I call *man-made*. These diseases are largely caused by an individual's lifestyle. To blame them on genetics or bad genes is valid only up to an extent. However, as you will read in this book, even a person's genetic makeup can be worked upon, altered, or influenced by lifestyle changes. In other words, "man-made" is dependent largely on the lifestyle of each person.

Foremost among my prescriptions for a healthy lifestyle is diet. I am a living example of someone who had numerous significant, painful, and discomforting health problems, and yet I overcame these largely because of thoughtful changes in my eating habits (healthy and tasty). By the same token, the important role of exercise for a healthy life cannot be emphasized enough.

It's not easy to change one's lifestyle, and it can't be done overnight. By taking tiny steps toward modifying one's habits, it becomes simpler to incorporate changes into one's daily life, and soon they become the new norm.

Some readers may never encounter a point of inflection (or reflection) that prompts them to change their lifestyle, as it happened to me post-surgery. However, one thing is certain: we live in uncertain times when many things are beyond our control. If there is one thing that we can control, it is the state of our hearts and our well-being. This book will enable you to improve *the quality of your heart, health, and your life,* even as we continue to face an uncertain future.

Up to the age of sixty-one, I was my biggest impediment to progress, and then I became my biggest change agent. I changed my attitude and beliefs, and adopted healthy eating, regular exercise, positivity, and meditation. Now at the age of seventy-three, I am living a life of purpose and of peace and contentment, doing everything I love.

I invite you to do so too.

Akil Taher

1

DOCTORS MAKE THE WORST PATIENTS

*You have no idea of what a poor opinion I have of myself, and
how little I deserve it.*

—W. S. GILBERT

IN 2003, A fifty-six-year-old physician, albeit successful and well-
respected in the medical community, had failed his first and
most important relationship in life—*he had failed his body, mind,
and spirit.*

Success had led to physical inactivity and vanity. He had seduced
his body with the indolent pleasure of being a couch potato. The only
exercise he got was his eye muscles staring at the treadmill. He would
say to himself, "Whenever you feel like exercise, lie down until the feeling abates."

I knew the doctor intimately. He enjoyed putting people down
because it validated his image of the wise guy. He took pride in winning
arguments, even if it meant making sarcastic quips and comebacks to
shut others up. Also, he would zone out if he were listening to something
he didn't want to hear. This didn't go down well with most of his friends.

The doctor was a party animal who indulged in compulsive

overeating, even though he was born with a genetic predisposition to heart and kidney disease, stroke, and diabetes. At the back of his mind he believed that *a doctor is a privileged class that knows it all,* and he relied on its omnipotent allies, science and medicine, for any effective cure or treatment. So, he could enjoy the finer things in life and feast on the best foods without worrying about the susceptibility of genes. He also dismissed various alternative practices, such as yoga, meditation, deep breathing, and spirituality, as a waste of time.

Being an eloquent communicator, he was a speaker for several pharmaceutical enterprises, including Pfizer, one of the world's largest pharmaceutical companies. Invited to speak in Birmingham, Alabama, the physician engaged in moderate social drinking with some attendees after the speaking engagement. On his way back home to Gadsden (an hour away from Birmingham), the doctor was stopped by a police officer for speeding.

The officer asked the doctor for his license and insurance papers, which he promptly handed over to the cop. The physician admitted to the speeding offense, yet his tone of his voice, the intent behind his words, epitomized the entitlement that comes with power, as if he were actually saying, "C'mon, don't waste my time. Just give me a ticket and be done with."

The unwarranted indifference obviously irked the police officer, who asked the doctor if he'd been drinking. The physician said, "Social drinking and no more."

The officer told the doctor to get out of the car and gave him the customary finger-to-nose and walk-and-turn sobriety test. The physician passed the test easily but still got a speeding ticket, doubtless because of his cavalier attitude.

In his relentless pursuit of recognition, the physician had worked hard to gain respect and appreciation in the community. The trade-off was that he couldn't give his family the attention and time it needed. After a long day at work, he came home fatigued, so tired and mentally drained that even talking to his wife and the kids felt like a chore. Each day after getting home, he would have a quiet dinner with the family and then go to bed. This became a routine.

The paradox of being an influential communicator in public but inept with his own family was playing out in the doctor's life. Here was a man who communicated only intermittently with his family, and yet exerted influence as an adept speaker.

While I loved the physician dearly, I was beginning to lose respect for him. An educated, curious, and financially savvy medical practitioner who had risen above the hardships of his early immigrant life in the United States, who worked arduously to build a better future for his family and himself, could not see the folly of his intemperate lifestyle and conceited mindset. The doctor had become blinded by his vanity in his expertise and the single-minded chase of recognition and respect ... *and I'm not ashamed to admit that this physician was ME.*

I had risked everything for the American dream. Unlike most immigrant doctors of Indian descent, I moved to the United States when I was almost forty years old. I had worked in Bahrain for eleven years with local American, British, and Australian doctors before I made America my home. I got my family practice certification from the American University of Beirut and was then a preceptor for the university's family practice residency program.

I was also involved in the opening of the first medical school in the Gulf region, the College of Medicine and Medical Sciences in the Arabian Gulf University (AGU) in Bahrain, where I taught medical students.

I was an experienced physician, but the move to the United States meant I had to start all over and rebuild my life from scratch. My overseas medical experience didn't mean much in the United States. I also had to complete medical residency training in order to practice as a physician.

My wife, Nafisa, jocularly remarked at the joint graduation party she threw for my son and me, "My husband, Akil, is the oldest resident to graduate from a family-practice residency program, and my son, Nikhil, is the youngest medical-school graduate in his class."

I was glad the residency training was over because for an experienced overseas physician, lining up a residency in the States was far from easy. I was prepared to start over, but forty (my age) is not a good number for program directors. They look for younger doctors who they believe can stand the pressure of working twelve to eighteen hours a day. In my mind, I did fit the bill because I was used to working long and unpredictable hours. But most of the fifty family-practice residency programs I applied for felt otherwise. Only six called me for an interview.

I remember going to New York for one of those interviews. The program director jokingly said, "I don't think you'll be able to keep up with the other residents, and besides you're overqualified. In fact, you're older than me."

I looked him square in the eye and said, "You'll never know until you give me a chance."

When I launched my practice as a physician, I was forty-five years old. I had a lot of catching up to do with immigrant doctors who were my age or slightly older and had come to the United States ten or fifteen years earlier. They were better placed than I because I had made America my home later than they.

I was now part of a hierarchical structure where my worth depended on my medical experience and specialization. I had the medical skills and the competence, but not the social network of the medical fraternity. I was treated as an inferior because I didn't have the same experience as other United States doctors did.

Respect and recognition always mattered to me more than money. I wanted to belong here. And to do so, I had to prove my worth and earn respect all over again, this time in the United States.

The pursuit of respect and admiration became my single-minded goal. This was one of the reasons I turned to public speaking and became a speaker for several pharmaceutical companies. Speaking helped me build credibility and establish expertise.

After years of diligent practice, I was now riding high because, in my mind, I had attained the respect I deserved and an upper-class status.

Success often breeds arrogance. Arrogance makes us feel powerful, but it also feeds ignorance. You can't see what's coming, or what you don't know can hurt you. Ignorance has a price. My blind spots were about to make me easy prey. And little did I know that a trip to London would be the beginning of the worst phase of my life.

In the summer of 2003, I went to London to visit a close friend. Early one morning, I decided to go for a walk in Hyde Park. Four minutes into the walk, I felt chest discomfort radiating to my right shoulder, accompanied by lightheadedness. I stopped and rested for a while. I continued walking and BOOM! Two hundred forty-two seconds later (I timed it), I got the same feeling in my chest. Being a physician, I knew in my mind it was angina, but my heart rejected it.

I didn't want to believe that a doctor who is supposed to be healthy is *not*. And yet when it started to sink in that all was not well, I was scared stiff. Apart from the fact that I was in a foreign country, I was no longer in control of my life. The very next day, I left for the US.

Upon my return home, I spent the first night tossing and turning under the covers. Fear gripped me and was choking the life out of me. Agitated and confused, my thoughts were running riot inside my tormented head, colliding with one another.

I was at war with myself, in heated conflict and denial. It was agonizing. I thought of every possible chest pain not related to the heart. I wasn't behaving rationally, going to great lengths to avoid accepting that my chest pain was linked to heart disease. For the first time, I had information aversion and wished I were not a doctor. *I knew too much that was unpleasant.*

The next day, I went to the local gym with reluctance and eyed the treadmills for a while. I told myself, "You lazy bones, you've never used your gym membership." Eventually, I mustered up the courage to get on the treadmill. I started slow, gradually transitioning to a brisk walk. For a while, everything went well. I was overjoyed, and started to jog. A few minutes later, I felt again the heaviness in my chest and a dull ache in my right shoulder. Super scared, I hit the big red knob, turning off the treadmill abruptly. I lost my balance and almost fell. Tears welled up, but I didn't want to show my weakness to fellow gym goers. A young man asked me if I was okay. I said, "Yes, it's just my allergies acting up."

It was time to get a stress test. The test turned out positive. The next step was to get an angiogram. The angiogram showed triple coronary artery blockages. I had a choice between open-heart (bypass) surgery or inserting stents into the clogged arteries. I was plagued by an acute rush of fear and unwilling for anyone to open me up. So I chose stents.

The stenting for two of my arteries had to be done on the same day, but during the procedure, I had a cardiac arrest. They had to postpone, putting off the second stent to the next day. I had to be shocked (emergency electric cardioversion) to get my stopped heart beating again. The next morning, I saw the red paddle burns on my chest along with hair loss. I joked with the nurses, saying, "I don't have to go to the beach now to get a tan."

I laughed to avoid crying, because I was horrified to see the paddle burns and the hair loss.

Seventy-two hours after the stents procedure I was back at work … the paramountcy of the work ethic. I had no chest pain but was very unhappy. While I was attentive to my patients' needs and carried out my professional responsibilities properly, all was not well in my personal life. I was perennially anxious and dispirited. I preferred to be alone, locked in bouts of silence, staring into space without any thought or purpose. These empty moments of staring into nothingness were born from the trauma of a doctor turning into a patient.

I hardly ate. As a result my abdomen would often growl loudly, embarrassing me at times when I was with patients. Nights were really tough. Tossing and turning, waking up with fear, and night sweats were commonplace. And the mornings were no better. By the time I finished putting clothes on to go to work, I experienced a constant lack of energy and fatigue. All of these dark energies were causes for concern. I was slowly disintegrating because at the back of my mind, I was carrying the burden that I had failed my family. I needed help, and Nafisa convinced me to see a psychiatrist.

It's often said that doctors are the worst patients, and it is difficult for doctors to admit they have become a patient. We think it is a stigma and are embarrassed to admit our illness. Disease and illness happen to other people, not us. We believe that we are at the top of the power hierarchy, over patients, sickness, and disease, and our extensive medical knowledge in preventing or curing illness makes us infallible. We forget that, like our patients, we are only human.

Doctors know how to treat pain, but it is difficult for them to understand the precise extent of pain or comprehend a patient's agony because they have largely experienced only one side of medicine—as doctors, not as patients. This also leads us to believe we are immune to any medical ailment or disease. And because I knew the precursors and causes of heart disease, it was unfathomable to me that I was a patient afflicted with a heart disorder … and yet the bitter truth was that I, a medical practitioner, was ill, and my body needed repair.

In my mind, my angst was heightened because my medical expertise had deserted me when I required it the most. And because I wasn't religious or spiritual, I couldn't find deeper meaning in my predicament or experience a sense of personal growth while living with a weaker heart.

The distance between the patient and the doctor had disappeared. The physician had become a patient. The audacity of invincibility had been shattered. I felt powerless. Something I had never imagined in my wildest dreams was happening to me. The impregnable doctor was now the difficult patient … and he was going to prove the adage that doctors make the worst patients.

The next five years were agonizing. I became a chronic complainer because I was consumed by fear-filled thoughts. Poor listening adversely affected my personal relationships. With my patients, I was an active listener, but with family and friends, I was impulsive and impatient. This alienated some of my dearest friends, hurt the feelings of my loved ones, and unwittingly wounded my spirit as well. Also, the constant feelings of panic and hopelessness, as if death were looming over me, took a toll on my mental health. Yet amidst all the stormy commotion in my life, there was a positive: I tried to do something to change my self-destructive disposition. But did it work?

I attended Deepak Chopra's seminar on improving the well-being of body, mind, and spirit. I also attended Dean Ornish's program for reversing heart disease, which consisted of following his *Eat More, Weigh Less* diet. Although this program has been successful for many people in improving their overall health, it didn't work for me. At that point, my mind hadn't come to terms with accepting the dietary recommendations, and so my heart wasn't in it. Simply put, I was a walking zombie.

Although I attempted to change my eating habits, I couldn't let go of my negative emotions and feelings. This affected my health in several ways. And when it rains, it pours.

Sinus infections and bronchitis made regular visits. Chronic constipation troubled me. Fissures and hemorrhoids added to my discomfort; and because I had severe diverticulitis, I was hospitalized twice with colon perforation. Not to forget the medication they gave me led to mouth ulcers for many years. I was now plagued with insurmountable health problems.

I was giving up on life. I believed I wasn't going to survive the ordeal of my body's many weaknesses and that I was going to die. Psychological distress and concern for the financial well-being of my family were giving me sleepless nights. I decided to streamline my finances and sold some of my assets to secure my family's financial future.

My efforts to better myself comprised of dietary modifications, financial restructuring, and superficial changes to my angst-ridden temperament. I thought these adjustments were adequate, but when the mending does not address the real problem, the efforts may seem impressive but are wasted.

I had a multitude of problems. My heart wasn't in it, for real. I wasn't taking my medications on a regular basis and the nonmedicated stents were not working. I had fallen prey to negative thinking that had drained my joy of the beautiful life I had created. Most importantly, the time had come for me to pay: to pay for abusing my body, mind, and spirit, to pay for my arrogance in my expertise, to pay for my caustic tongue, and to pay for the intoxication of success. So, it came as no surprise that in 2009, I had restenosis of my coronary arteries (a gradual re-narrowing of a coronary artery after it has been treated with angioplasty and stenting) and had to have open-heart (bypass) surgery at St. Michael's Medical Center in New Jersey.

A sixty-one-year-old physician was left with only one chance to resurrect to a new life.

2

ADVERSITY CAN BE
YOUR BEST FRIEND OR
YOUR WORST ENEMY

Adversity has the effect of eliciting talents, which in prosperous circumstances would have lain dormant.

—HORACE

M Y HEART, THE essence of my being, the center of my desires and pleasures, hopes and dreams, feelings and emotions, was under siege. Twenty-two years after immigrating to the United States, I had experienced an "epic" blow. The open-heart surgery to repair the damage in my heart was to be performed at St. Michael's Medical Center in New Jersey. Was this the beginning of an overly cautious life?

I had never been content with an ordinary existence. Being normal wasn't good enough for me. I hadn't taken various risks and overcome many struggles to have my life come to an abrupt standstill, devoid of all adventure, because of a bypass surgery. I wasn't prepared to lead an unimaginative life. I wasn't ready to end up in the rocking chair. I would wither away and die faster if I didn't do anything significant because my genetics weren't about mere existence. Thankfully, there was a flip side to my obstinate vanity. Determination ran deep in my veins.

I knew that to restore my life to my normal, I had to embrace the super normal. I had to abandon the ordinary by taking my own journey to the extraordinary. And I had to reincarnate into a new life and to stay true to the meaning of my first name, Akil—*the wise.*

These thoughts, hidden in the deepest recesses of my mind, together with the lingering effects of anesthesia may have led me to promise the nursing staff at the intensive care unit of St. Michael's Medical Center that if my post-operative recovery went well, I would run at least a half marathon (13.1 miles) in a year's time. They must have thought I was out of my mind. But that casual comment became the defining moment of my life.

Sometimes poor health or bad times can elicit a transformation that otherwise wouldn't happen. My open-heart surgery in August 2009 redefined the path of my life. I had hit rock bottom, and I hit it hard. I knew how to deal with everyday struggles, but nobody ever taught me how to overcome a major setback. I knew no one who could pull me out of this tailspin. I had to do it myself.

After the surgery, I reflected on my life. I could either continue with my immoderate lifestyle and face the catastrophic consequences, or I could do something worthwhile with my life. I chose the latter.

Obstinacy was replaced by determination, arrogance by introspection, and negativity with positivity.

I wasn't going to change, I was going to transform. I wasn't going to be a burden to my supportive and remarkable family. I was going to be the husband and dad my family could be proud of. In my earlier avatar, I had been self-absorbed. In my rebirth, I was going to be a beacon of hope for senior citizens navigating the winter of their lives, or the darkest passage of their lives. Thus, a sixty-one-year-old physician, husband, and dad was born again. Life had given him a second chance.

Until now, I had merely pursued materialism without purpose, and that had left me unhealthy and unfulfilled. I was now going to take a big step to bring meaningful purpose to my life.

I don't know whether it was my belief, the amazing care I was given, or both, but my recovery was remarkable. The third day after my triple bypass surgery, I was back on my feet. Not just on my feet, but on the treadmill. I felt great. Even with the excruciating pain that accompanied the dreaded coughing, I didn't take pain medications. I was happier in physical pain than in the emotional agony I had undergone in the last five years. My spirit was untamed.

I had seen many of my patients go from heart surgery to the rocking chair. I knew that depression and inactivity were common among heart-surgery patients. The fear that exertion will trigger or cause a heart attack is so pronounced, it can impede recovery or lead to physical inactivity. And physical inertia increases the level of depression.

To avoid being a victim of depression, I had to make a lifestyle change and do something constructive and therapeutic. To truly live, I had to dramatically alter the conventional script adopted by most elderly heart patients. And even though I was scared, I decided to do what I feared most—*strenuous exercise.* For a sedentary slob like me, vigorous exercise was going to be accompanied by stiffness and soreness.

Yet while I was improving my lifestyle, I had not improved the quality of my life. To do so, I had to improve and nourish my body, mind, and soul. I had to start something new and impactful. Thanks to the famous Irish middle-distance runner Noel Carroll, who once said, "Running is the classical road to self-consciousness, self-awareness, and self-reliance," I was motivated to put on my running shoes. And to make the most of the second chance life had given me, I decided I would run a half marathon within the year. The promise to the nurses who had generously assisted me during my surgery served as the inducement.

My idea of running a half marathon was initially met with resistance from my family, who thought I was crazy, perhaps going through some kind of midlife crisis.

I replied, "This is my last chance to reform and lead a fulfilling and happier life. I'm not going to screw it up."

My kids said, "Your genetics are bad, you can't fight your genes."

"Yes, I do have bad heart genes. But I can't use that as a crutch."

I assured my family that I would outsmart my genes through nutrition and healthy lifestyle changes, and that I would not jeopardize my health by rushing into intensive running or rigorous training. They reluctantly agreed.

I took baby steps to running. First walking, then jogging, and then running. There was no set plan. I did not read any books about how to run half marathons. I went to the park behind the Sears in our small town of Gadsden, Alabama, and took small steps each day that made exercising enjoyable, not frustrating or exhausting. And I ensured I exercised alone so that I could tailor the workout to my body's needs. I had my own goals, and I could go as soft, hard, or short as I wanted. There were no hills to climb, and runners had told me that if I could complete nine miles, that would suffice. For the last 4.1 miles, I could rely on adrenaline-fueled enthusiasm, the atmosphere, and crowd support to get me across the line.

Independence is the classical outstanding character of the runner. It helped me to embrace solo running, enjoy being alone with my thoughts, and cherish the beauty of nature—the joyful sounds of chirping birds, the burbling of waterfalls, and the whispers of the trees as the wind blew through their branches. I was meditating with open eyes.

I could do some of my best thinking while running. I began to listen more to what my body was telling me. This enhanced my physical and mental well-being. My type A personality mellowed. I was now more peaceful, receptive, and a better listener. I also learned to compete with myself to better myself. This was radically different from previous years when I competed with peers in the medical fraternity for financial one-upmanship. I was now setting a bar for myself, and my goal was only to become a better version of myself.

Training was tough, but it was for a bigger purpose. I still remember my initial struggles with calf and back pain, as well as other body aches. My muscles were revolting since they had never done anything like this before. Nevertheless, I persisted, and the pain got better with continued running.

After every long run, I ate like a horse, but since I was eating better, my stomach was at peace. Once when I completed the customary nine miles, I took my brother-in-law—who was visiting from out of town—to a show in Birmingham. Overcome with tiredness, I not only slept through the whole show, my wife elbowed me in the side because I was snoring.

I spent six months in training and preparation to embark on a mission to run and transform my life. An ardent belief in a higher power, familial support, faith in myself, and an effective dietary change were instrumental in preparing me for the next big challenge of my life.

In April 2010, eight months after my triple bypass surgery, I ran my first half marathon. It was the 13.1-mile Nashville Country Music Half Marathon in Nashville, Tennessee. I had turned a serious setback into a comeback. The adventurous twists of my life had just begun.

Adversity can be your best friend or your worst enemy

Life, credit cards, and adversity come with expiration dates. Adversity is inevitable but temporary. Adversity can be your best friend or your worst enemy. That depends upon you. You can back down in the face of adversity and never bounce back, or you can go through it with courage, self-belief, and determination to discover your true potential and purpose. Take baby steps to overcome adversity. First walk, then jog, then run, and then you will cruise. That is how you turn adversity into a meaningful life.

3

MARATHONS AND MY RESURRECTION

Do the thing you fear most and the death of fear is certain.

—MARK TWAIN

My First Half Marathon in Nashville, Tennessee (April 2010)

I FINISHED MY FIRST half marathon in over three grueling hours. Eight months after my open-heart surgery, I completed the 13.1-mile Nashville Country Music Half Marathon in Nashville, Tennessee. It was one of the happiest moments of my life. I had given a befitting reply to my rebellious body, which during the preparation phase repeatedly said, "Why have you started doing all this at sixty-one? Don't you have better things to do?"

Six months of self-guided preparation devoid of warm-ups and cooldowns (stretching was the only warm-up), with flat-surface training done four to five times a week on a trail behind the Sears in our small town, and not being challenged by any hills (there were none to climb) did lack the rigors of training for a half marathon, yet to my determined mind, it was good enough to cross the first hurdle—the first nine miles. For the last 4.1 miles, I would tell myself, "I will walk or crawl if I have to." But even that sounded daunting.

A night before the half marathon, my wife and I drove to Nashville, which is about three hours from Gadsden. I went to bed around 9 p.m., but I couldn't sleep. I was a bundle of nerves. The dichotomy of excitement and fear was building. Will my enthused *new* heart spur me to cross the finish line, or would it give me dreaded chest pains and force me to abandon the race? Would I be able to get over the first hurdle, the nine miles? Would I be able to walk the last 4.1 miles?

Finally at about 2 a.m., I dozed off and had a very strange dream. I was representing the United States in the Olympics, and there were tears of joy as they placed the medal around my neck. I was singing the country's national anthem, *The Star-Spangled Banner* (of course, totally out of tune). At the back of my mind, I knew bigger things were waiting to happen in my life. Was this inexplicable dream a precursor to bigger celebratory events in my life? Only time would tell.

The morning did witness the continuation of the butterflies in my stomach. I was as nervous as a long-tailed cat in a room full of rocking chairs. I paced the hotel room, and once every hour, I used the bathroom. I don't remember eating anything that morning. I was caffeine-free jittery.

I had arrived in Nashville for one of the biggest challenges of my life. The moment of reckoning finally arrived. I was at the start line. I was tense, so I started slow. After about a mile or so, I saw a big hill. I tried to convince myself it was the only hill, but I was wrong. There were more. Not only had I not trained on hills, I hadn't known hills were going to be part of the half marathon.

My mediocre preparation and anxious mindset weren't going to help me finish the race. Until that moment, I had carried the burden of running a half marathon as if it were a huge undertaking. I had to change that overwhelming mindset, and fortunately, I did. I approached the half marathon with reckless abandon. The stress turned into positive energy. As the saying goes, "If you can't beat them, join them." That's exactly what I did. I started enjoying the experience and having fun. Finally, I had a smile on my face. For me, this was the turning point of the half marathon.

I took delight in the country music bands playing along the way.

People were cheering us, the participants. Some even offered me beer. Such generosity of spirit, and I will let you be the judge as to whether I accepted the malted beverage or not. I was so pumped up, enjoying the moment and taking everything in.

Suddenly, out of nowhere, there were thunderstorms, and it started to rain. By now, I had completed ten or eleven miles. I heard an announcement that they were going to cancel the race if lightning began. A lot of people abandoned the race. I did not.

I was on a high, reveling in nature's munificence and soaking in its grandeur. So I continued running. I didn't care if I finished or not. My attention was only my actions and not the outcome. You can't fight nature. Earlier, I would fight things that could not be changed, and now I had begun to accept those things. By now, this marked there was a big conversion in me.

I finished the half marathon in over three hours. It was demanding and enervating, but the exhilaration of achieving a seemingly insurmountable goal after bypass surgery outweighed my fatigue. Euphoria, catharsis, and an inexplicable inner peace gripped my body, mind, and spirit. The defining moment had arrived.

My body had overcome surgery, nerves, fear, aches, pains, bad genetics, and exhaustion to live up to the promise the man had made to the nursing staff at the intensive care unit of St. Michael's Medical Center: If his post-operative recovery went well, he would run at least a half marathon in a year's time. Well, he did fine, and ran the race eight months later.

My heart had *not* failed me. It physically and figuratively carried me to the finish line.

The Chicago Marathon
My First Full Marathon (October 2011)
The Marathon with a Purpose

Man fools himself. He prays for a long life, and he fears an old age.

—CHINESE PROVERB

For many, life begins at twenty-one, or twenty-five, or forty, or sixty. For me, it began at sixty-one and got better at sixty-three.

Life shouldn't stop after a major health crisis. We are all mortal and, therefore, subject to age, illness, and slowdown, but we have a powerful ally in an attribute that all of us possess, that is free and unlimited: willpower. And we must recognize the role that willpower or inner strength play in improving our health.

When we are purpose driven, enjoy or fall in love with our leisure pursuits, or our eyes open wide with excitement because our mission is lofty, we have more energy. We recover quickly from any illness or disease, and age becomes just a number.

We are capable of doing much more than we think we can do. We can safely push ourselves beyond what we believe are our physical limits when we feel challenged and excited by a meaningful project or endeavor. We can then reach the acme of our potential.

With this thought in mind, I decided to run a full marathon, the Chicago Marathon, and become a 0.5 percenter. That is, join the ranks of the *0.5 percent of the US population who have run a full marathon.*[1]

Having completed two half marathons (Nashville and Zooma Atlanta), I was now better prepared and able to appreciate the importance of consistent training, nutrition, warm-ups, and cooldowns. This time, I was far more professional and did my homework prudently. I read *The Marathon Method* by Tom Holland, *Born to Run* by Christopher McDougall, and *The Non-Runner's Marathon Trainer* by David A. Whitsett, Forrest A. Dolgener, and Tanjala Mabon Kole. I also wrote a letter to my friends on my sixty-third birthday, letting them know I intended to compete in the Chicago Marathon that October.

Unlike before my first half marathon, I completed fifteen minutes of stretching—which involved quads, hamstrings, glutes, hip flexors, abs, back, and calves—before I started my practice run. The stretching was followed by breathing exercises to gradually build up my lung capacity, a sure way to give me more wind for running. At least thirty minutes of breathing and stretching did improve my lung capacity and prevented muscle strain or workout injury.

After the practice run, I would walk for a quarter of a mile to cool down and then sit in the car. Earlier, my running had been restricted to the flat trail behind Sears in Gadsden, but now it included the roads, uphills, and downhills of Gadsden. I preferred running uphill because not only was it great for enhancing my stamina, it also built my leg muscles, which would augment my speed and make the final ten kilometers (6.2 miles) of a full marathon feel easier. I knew that uphill running also reduced the risk of shin splints, and because it required me to breathe harder, it increased my lung capacity.

After the open-heart surgery and before the first half marathon, I had gone to The Art of Living Foundation in Atlanta and attended several courses. That got me into yoga, meditation, and breathing techniques. I religiously practiced a yoga exercise, Surya Namaskar (sun salutation), that keeps the mind active and calm while strengthening the entire body.

I ate healthier with more of a vegetarian diet. I cut down on meat, dairy, and eggs, and harnessed myself up with a carbohydrate diet and a good breakfast. I felt more peaceful and receptive with this change in my diet and its emphasis on vegetables and grains.

The Chicago Marathon was the first time I was getting onto the big boys' field, so I hired an accomplished personal trainer, Stacey Garmon. My trainer saw something in me that I didn't. I couldn't fool her as she was a hard taskmaster.

Discipline was the key here, and an integrated strategy that comprised appropriate diet and nutrition, physical and mental training (the stretching and breathing exercises, running, yoga, and meditation) slowly got me from nine miles to eighteen to twenty miles. And through all this, I was up at five every day, and would then complete all my training before leaving for work at eight.

I did all my practice runs as suggested by marathon gurus. But I must confess, it wasn't easy. There were days when my knees hurt. Osteoarthritis ran in my family, and I had to do long-distance running now. My dad and uncles had balloons for knees. My diverticulitis (inflammation of pouches in the wall of the colon) would flare up occasionally, as did the ache from previously fractured vertebrae. My sixty-three years were catching up on me.

There were days when it was cold outside, and I would rather be snuggled up in the house with my wife and dog. There were even days when I did not have the energy to do a "light" four-mile run, but I ran through it all. None of my injuries was going to stop me from running because each time I ran, I forgot my woes, and the elation of running outweighed the pain. The passion for running was so intense, the pain became secondary. And I never missed running or exercising because of snow, even though Gadsden saw only a few days of snowfall.

The love of running and accepting challenges notwithstanding, the deeper purpose of running the Chicago Marathon was to raise money. Since cardiovascular disease (heart disease) is the number one killer in America and I fell victim to it, I committed to raising money for the American Heart Association (AHA). I wasn't a seasoned fundraiser, but I did my best and single-handedly raised close to $11,000. These funds went toward prevention of heart disease, emergency care, cardiac surgeries, and other forms of treatment.

This was my first full marathon, and I wanted to give it my all. I trained hard, but as luck would have it, I had a problem with my left foot. I had a dropped second metatarsal (acute pain in the ball of your foot), and it was equivalent to walking with a marble in your foot. I consulted with a physical therapist, orthopedist, and acupuncturists, and the general consensus was that I should use metatarsal pads, which would make my feet feel better and partially relieve the discomfort.

Thankfully, I had been told that further running wasn't going to make it worse. I rested my foot for three weeks and was then back in training. During this period, I didn't have an iota of doubt that I would run and finish the marathon, perhaps because I had prepared earnestly and felt fighting fit.

Since this was my first big race, my children decided to join me. We reached Chicago a day before the race. Everyone went out to dinner, but I stayed back to mentally prepare for the race. I had a quick pasta dish at the hotel restaurant and called it an early night.

When I woke at 5 a.m., I began the ritual that I follow before every major event. I start by drinking a large glass of lukewarm water, followed by a cup of coffee, shave, shower, and a light breakfast of toast and a banana.

At the start line, I was ready and raring to go. Soon, I would be a marathoner. It was hot and humid by Midwest standards, with the temperature rising to 77°F as the race progressed. Runners were taking off their shirts, pouring water over their body. I spotted a pregnant lady, and on her T-shirt were printed the words: "I have my OB/GYN permission to run this marathon."

Talking about marathon pregnancy and its marvels ... Amber Miller, of Westchester, Illinois, completed the Chicago Marathon with a half-run, half-walk approach, beating her husband's time, and then gave birth to a baby daughter about seven hours later.

"Baby's first marathon," cried one supporter.

"Go, pregnant lady," cheered another.

A marathon of contrasting destinies. The circle of life and death was witnessed in the same race. Greensboro (North Carolina) Fire Department Captain William Caviness died, collapsing just yards from the finish line. Tragic, indeed.

I ran this marathon with ease. As I entered the last stretch of the race—the final two to three miles—I hit my second wind. That new burst of energy, so much energy, carried me to what I term my epic finish line. The memories of early-morning training, days of aches, soreness, and pains came back in a rush of nostalgia. The euphoric feeling of accomplishment and pride was coupled with tears of ecstasy.

I crossed the finish line and hugged my wife and children. I was now a *marathoner*. The sixty-three-year-old had completed the Chicago Marathon in five hours and twenty-eight minutes.

The card I got from my children:

Dear Dad,

Words cannot explain how proud we are of you.

You ran a freaking marathon you crazy man! 26.2 miles is no joke and training for 26.2 miles is no joke either! You made it happen! We are inspired by your dedication and commitment and hope to take a note from your lesson book. We love you so much!

Persistence
is a big, fancy word for "never giving up."

Determination
is just another way of saying "no ifs, ands, or buts."

Courage
is about having to do what needs to be done.

The Boston Marathon
My Second Full Marathon (April 2014)
The Marathon for Solidarity

At this period of my life, some people talked about me being addicted to marathons. But I had a specific reason to run the Boston Marathon (the world's oldest annual marathon that dates back to 1897). I wanted to express support and solidarity with the citizens of Boston and the participants of the previous year's race, especially those who were injured. In 2013, in a dastardly act of terrorism, a bomb during the marathon killed three people and injured more than 260 others. I felt a strong call to unite with them through running, particularly with the families of the afflicted.

The 2014 Boston Marathon had about 36,000 registered participants, second only to the 1996 race in the number of entries. The *Boston Globe* reported that over a million people were expected to line the marathon route to watch the race, twice the number that attended during a typical year.

"Many of us want to be there this year not merely to run or watch a road race, but to reclaim a beloved Boston event, one that always saw the city bursting with early spring fever and civic pride. People want to show the bombers that they failed, that the city will not be cowed," wrote Patrick Kennedy in a *Boston Globe* article that was published on March 23, 2014. Kennedy captured the precise sentiments that echoed within me.

The Boston Marathon is considered the holy grail of all marathons. I trained hard and vigorously for at least six months for the marathon (far more than I did for the Chicago Marathon) to improve my completion time to a respectable four hours and thirty minutes.

This time, I started every morning with an energy blend that included broccoli, celery, an apple, spinach, and carrot, followed by breathing and stretching exercises, yoga and meditation. I was now primarily a vegetarian, eating fish only on rare occasions. In spite of my preparations for exercising and keeping to a healthy diet, I hit a snag in my carefully planned routine. As the seers have often said, "Man plans, Mother Nature laughs." Five weeks prior to the marathon, I tore a calf muscle (the soleus muscle, one of the three muscles located in the calf) during one of my practice running sessions. It is a rare injury that happens to only about 5 percent of runners.

I was in the midst of a long sixteen-mile run. It was in Gadsden where there are 5K and 10K markers for the local races. I was hoping to do two 10Ks and finish off with a 5K.

Running alone, I started off great, running at ease and picking up speed till I had completed nine miles. Suddenly, I felt pain in my calf muscle. My first thought was that it could be a muscle spasm, so I continued. But the pain would not let up. I stopped, took a deep breath, and started walking. The pain got worse, and soon I was limping. *Had I torn a muscle?* I asked myself.

I did not want to think about it anymore. Taking a shortcut, I barely managed to limp back to my car. I was angry and hurt. I took off the shoe and threw it at the car, blaming the roads, the shoes, and even my own genetics.

Under the advice of my orthopedist and radiologist, I decided not to run the marathon. *I was going to walk the race.* A setback wasn't going to deter me from participating. David Ellis, a physical therapist at Gadsden Regional Medical Center, and Stacey Garmon, my personal trainer, worked zealously, and they were instrumental in getting me to the point where at least walking the 26.2-mile race was a possibility. I told myself that I would walk the 26.2 miles, even if it meant walking well into the next day. I would give it my all to honor the victims of the Boston Marathon bombing.

The Boston Marathon begins on Main Street in Hopkinton, a small suburb west of Boston, and weaves through six other cities before reaching the finish line in Copley Square.

Runners from Boston are loaded into buses to be taken to Hopkinton. Our driver missed the exit, and it took quite some time to get back on the right exit. We were all anxious, afraid we would not reach the starting line in time, even as most of us were also dying to pee. We reached Hopkinton but still had to walk to where the race began. Seeing long lines at the bathrooms, most of us ran to the first open space and relieved ourselves.

I joined the Boston Marathon participants on what was a cold April day. The festive atmosphere rivaled the one I had experienced in Chicago. I expected some pain as I started off, but since I felt no discomfort, I cautiously slow jogged the first ten miles, spurred by the adrenaline rush and the spectators' encouraging cheers. Much of the credit for my feeling good and for the relatively pain-free jog goes to David's magic touch and Stacey's patient effort.

I followed David's advice and stretched my left calf muscle after each mile. I repeated this until I completed the first ten miles. After that, the damaged calf muscle started acting up, although not in any serious manner.

My awareness of the subdued but nagging pain would have made no difference to my jogging under ordinary circumstances, but Nafisa had told me not to come home if I injured myself. Of course, she didn't mean that literally, but I did not want to listen to her telling me "I told you so" or for her to face the prospect of having to nurse an injured man back to health. I decided not to take the chance of seriously hurting myself again, and I transitioned from the slow jog to a slow trot-walking combination. Even though my slower pace should have increased my time, I saved time overall because I didn't have to stretch my calf muscles after every mile.

I had worn a knit toboggan at the start of the race to keep warm, but I took it off as it was getting too hot. With $20 in my pocket, I approached a stranger on the sidewalk and offered him money in exchange for his baseball hat. He was reluctant at first, but his girlfriend told him to hand it over to me. Not only that, but she refused to take the $20. As a parting shot, the man let me know that the hat had been his for ten years. "You better finish the race," he shouted at my back. In retrospect, his words were part of my motivation for finishing the race. I tried hard to find him after the race, went online, asked the authorities if they could help, but they all wanted his name. He made a difference that day, and I hope he gets to read this book.

Soldiering on, I made it to the seventeenth mile before my calf muscle began to ache. I was about to face one of the toughest parts of the course, Heartbreak Hill, the infamous incline considered by many as the most difficult challenge of the Boston Marathon course. Dealing with three hills right before it in Newton made Heartbreak Hill even more challenging.

Heartbreak Hill is a steep half mile at mile 20. The uphill didn't bother me. For me, the toughest part in a marathon is going down-hill because it is acutely uncomfortable for my quadriceps muscles. The downhill from the top of Heartbreak Hill to Cleveland Circle was not only a grueling test of endurance, it was also anguishing. I felt like my quadriceps were being ripped apart. This drained my energy levels as well.

This stretch was even tougher for me because I'd had no actual marathon training for the five weeks before the race. Everything hurt. My muscles burned like they had been lit on fire, and my bones ached deep into the marrow. But the screaming and cheering spectators egged me on, helping me lean on my mental prowess to make it through the formidable hill.

As I entered the home stretch, I spotted Nafisa and gained the much-needed inspiration to finish what I had started. I could now taste victory lying just two miles away. I was at the last remnants of my energy, but I willed my body to keep moving forward. It didn't matter whether I walked, ran, or crawled to that coveted line.

However, I stayed upright and completed the marathon in five hours and forty-eight minutes, proud for completing the race when only a few weeks back, I'd had doubts about even participating. At the same time, for just a split second, I felt disappointed that I hadn't completed the marathon in my self-allocated time period of four hours and thirty minutes.

People around me put my disappointment on the back burner, thumping my back and praising my accomplishment. I realized I was being too severe on myself and felt gratified that I had finished the race in spite of a torn calf muscle. Someday, I thought, this would make an interesting story to tell my grandson Kai.

Standard Chartered Mumbai Marathon
India's Largest Annual Marathon (January 2016)
The Marathon for Gratitude and Heart Philanthropy

I became an accomplished marathoner, but I mainly ran marathons that had some meaning to me. To this end, I could not help but set my eyes on the Standard Chartered Mumbai Marathon in India, considered to be Asia's largest marathon in terms of participation and magnitude.

I was now sixty-seven years old and realized I could not go on running marathons forever. To me, this would be a fitting way to retire, as I was born in Mumbai (the City of Dreams) and had great memories of my childhood in a metropolis that never tires nor sleeps, and has a big heart. I had a deep sense of gratitude for Mumbai and India. It was now my turn to give back to the city and country that gave me so much.

In January 2016, I traveled to India to run the marathon. To lend their support, my daughter, Anushka, and my niece, Urvashi, decided to run with me.

Another reason I was participating in the Standard Chartered

Mumbai Marathon was to raise funds for the Bombay Medical Aid Foundation, a philanthropic organization dedicated to providing free medical services to those suffering from heart disease, particularly the underprivileged. I was fortunate to have been able to afford my open-heart surgery, but what about the underprivileged of India? My effort was a drop in the ocean, but for the city and the country that gave me the wings to fly, this was the least I could do.

I knew from experience that running a marathon in a busy and chaotic city like Mumbai would be diametrically different from any other half or full marathon I had run in the United States. I couldn't replicate the Mumbai marathon conditions while training in the United States, so I did what I thought would make for a smart preparation. I trained intensively for a few months in Gadsden, and then, because I go to Mumbai once a year, I also trained in Mumbai during July and August 2015 to acclimatize myself for the January 2016 marathon.

I stayed in South Mumbai at Nariman Point. From there, I would run all the way to the Hanging Gardens perched at the top of Malabar Hill, and then turn around and run back to Nariman Point, where my hotel was located. I did these practice runs, some in heavy rain (it was the monsoon season) about four or five times during my visit to Mumbai.

For an old pro who had run marathons before, these practice runs were a breeze. There was little physical strain, and I devoted most of my runs to soaking in the sights, sounds, and smells of the South Mumbai streets.

I saw health-conscious people of all ages walk every morning on the wide promenades at Marine Drive, Chowpatty Beach, Walkeshwar, and Malabar Hill. The older people were a delight to watch, their bonhomie uplifting my spirits as they walked, talked, waved, smiled, and laughed with those around them. Each day, I felt blessed by the Prasāda (a religious offering or consecrated food) given to me and other joggers, walkers, and bystanders by people who combined their early morning walk with a visit to the revered Babulnath Temple near Chowpatty Beach.

The sight of South Mumbai's skyline, the sound of the waves of the Arabian Sea crashing against the boulders placed there as a deterrent to flooding, and the cool breeze that ran through my hair were uplifting and soulful. These led me to experience a meditative serenity with open eyes.

On the day of the Standard Chartered Mumbai Marathon, Sunday, January 17, 2016, the streets along the course were empty of the traffic snarls that India's most car-congested city is dubiously famous for, a testament to the efficiency of the organizers. All roads reserved for the race were closed and strictly policed, and there were no cars parked all along the course of the marathon.

All the participants were expected to convene at the historic Azad Maidan, a majestic sports ground located on twenty-five acres of land near the world's busiest train station, Chhatrapati Shivaji Terminus station. I was back in the country of my birth, and it felt poignant and nostalgic.

In US cities where marathons are held, things are calm and quiet during the wee hours of the morning on marathon day, but Mumbai was bursting with activity and noise. During my practice runs at Nariman Point, the smog and air pollution didn't affect my visibility or breath, but at Azad Maidan, both smog and air pollution were there to see and feel, so I knew I was starting with a disadvantage.

I was amazed to see the mammoth throng of runners; we were told it ranged between 40,000–45,000 people. The gigantic crowd had the flavor of inclusiveness in it. The elite, the wealthy, the celebrated, the middle class, and the underprivileged were going to run alongside each other. But this was India. In spite of the excellent preparations for the marathon, one simply could not stop the thousands of people weaving through the closed streets of Flora Fountain to get to Azad Maidan. For the runners, it was time-consuming and unnerving to navigate through the jaywalkers. Yet an air of eager anticipation and vibrant energy filled the air … all waiting to start and complete the marathon.

The race commenced at 05:40 a.m., so we had to run nearly an hour in the dark. It was around 64°F at the start line, but by 8:30 it was quite warm. The roads were not paved, and potholes were commonplace. I was worried about injury. Instead of looking ahead, I had to keep an eye to the ground, for stepping into a pothole could have dire consequences. To my surprise, the potholes didn't bother my daughter, Anushka. She just flew off.

To their credit, the organizers had done a terrific job plotting the route of the marathon, taking in many of the most classical and celebrated sites of the island city, particularly of South Mumbai. Chhatrapati Shivaji Terminus, Flora Fountain, Marine Drive, Chowpatty Beach, Babulnath Temple, Haji Ali Mosque, Mahalaxmi Race Course, the Nehru Centre, Siddhivinayak Temple, Rajiv Gandhi Sea Link bridge), and more. The course included all these iconic sights. I had visited or frequently passed by most of these historic locations while growing up in Mumbai in the '50s, '60s, and early '70s.

As South Mumbai consists mainly of reclaimed ground, I knew it was largely flat, barring the Peddar Road hill between Chowpatty Beach and Haji Ali Beach, which is roughly 0.6 miles up and then down. For me, who had encountered longer hills in the United States, particularly Heartbreak Hill in Boston, this small stretch was not much of a bother.

The beauty of the marathon was the heterogeneity of the challenges that accompanied it. You could either enjoy it or crib about it. The early morning cloud of smog and air pollution that enveloped the skies did irritate my eyes, but that paled in comparison to the happiness I experienced running while the Mumbai skyline was waking up.

From the start of the race, I wanted to keep an eye on my niece, Urvashi, because this was her first marathon, and she would need me to lend a word or two of encouragement to complete the race. At some point in the race, her toe started to bleed and hurt because she was wearing the wrong shoes. It is actually called a jogger's toe, caused by wearing shoes that are too small for you. But she braved it out and continued running.

To help Urvashi, I would go forward and then wait for her to catch up, and then I would run beside her for a while. At times, I would also go to the back to see if she was doing fine. I tried different things to ensure she continued, and to her credit she responded with dogged determination to carry on, despite the risk of serious injury from wearing the wrong running shoes.

While portable bathrooms were placed on the peripheries along the entire stretch of the race, the gargantuan number of participants meant that the long lines and waits for bathroom use would take up additional time. I had an enlarged prostate, so running without easy and swift access to a restroom was tough, truly an ordeal. So, I restricted my fluids to minimize the need to use the bathroom. That is the worst thing to do in a marathon because you will get spasms around eighteen or nineteen miles; and by the last few miles, I cringed from the intense pain in both my calf muscles. But the pain couldn't stop me from carrying on for a charity dear to my heart. On that day, my mind and spirit was stronger than my aching body.

The camaraderie of the participants and the collective espousal of the supporters was something I had not encountered in my previous marathon runs. The onlookers were clapping, cheering, and chanting collective and inspirational slogans in English, Hindi, and Marathi (the official language of the state of Maharashtra, of which Mumbai is the capital), while upbeat Bollywood music played in the background. "C'mon, let's go on. Don't give up," they said, urging us on.

As a sign of respect for elders, younger runners gave me way while running, and volunteers offered me water at regular intervals, remarking, "Uncle, would you like some water?" If I stopped for water, a younger runner who had already seen me slow down would hand his or her water to me, asking me to drink before he or she did, out of respect for my age.

The young volunteers and runners did not address me by my first name or affix a *Mr.* to my last name, but affectionately called me *Uncle.* In India, it is a sign of disrespect if you call someone vastly older than you by name.

The race was well supported, with bottled water provided every half a mile, not to forget wet sponges and orange juice at various stops. Volunteers along the course came out to support and rekindle our spirits, often with bananas and cookies (biscuits). Police lined the entire route in the light of terrorist threats. I saw a few medics on standby along the way too.

The final stretch along Marine Drive and into Chhatrapati Shivaji Terminus felt like a carnival, a remarkable medley of cheering supporters, photographers, and bandstands with performers, musicians, and marching bands.

It wasn't about who you were or the brand of shoes you wore, it was about the zest of participation. The age diversity of the participants was remarkable. The twelve-year-olds mingled with the septuagenarians as they ran for different reasons. Some participants ran to show solidarity for the city they owed everything to; some as a hobby; some to shed that extra weight; some to stay fit; and others to raise awareness about the pressing need to make lifestyle changes and get more health conscious, even as India, battles with heart disease that is now its deadliest killer. And then there were some participants who ran barefoot. I had the opportunity of meeting one such person, and he told me it was his dream to run a marathon, but he could not afford shoes. So he was running barefoot.

The moderately humid weather, the overwhelming crowd, the excruciating discomfort of holding my bladder for hours with an enlarged prostate owing to long bathroom lines and waits, the high security that cordoned off easily accessible areas, and the need for three eyes—one for the potholed roads, one to keep Urvashi in sight, and the other to enjoy the collective bonhomie of the slogan-chanting marathon participants—all combined to get me finally to the finish line.

Given the enormous magnitude of the marathon and the heightened security, it was never going to be easy to find our way from the finish line to the car that would drive us to our hotel. It took us two hours of jostling our way out of the disbursing and excited crowd to locate our car, and that precisely why I call it the most vibrant marathon of my life. There were moments of extreme uneasiness, but no moment was ever dull. Moments of despair were overpowered by moments of generosity and graciousness that are mine to keep for life. I would recommend every marathoner run the Mumbai Marathon (now sponsored by the TATA Group) once in his or her lifetime.

I was now a marathoner on two different continents, a marathoner who was honored by the presence and completion of the race by his daughter and niece, and a marathoner who had fulfilled his promise, purpose, and passion. The last long race of my life was special, meaningful, colorful, and it ended where my life began: Mumbai, the city with a big heart that gave me my first and only love, my first medical degree, my first true friends, and the opportunity for me to celebrate my homecoming as a full marathoner.

Then there's the indomitable 67-year-old Akil Taher who has landed from the US to run his last full marathon in Mumbai. For someone who ran his first marathon six years ago and eight months after an open-heart surgery, Taher's key offering is his spirit, apart from supporting the Bombay Medical Aid Foundation.

So wrote Mohua Das in an article published in the *Times of India* (Mumbai edition) on January 13, 2016. The *Times of India* is the largest-selling English-language daily newspaper in India.

Thank you, Mumbai, thank you, India, thank you, Bombay Medical Aid Foundation. You all have a special place in my heart.

Date with walks and thrive, not survive

Make dates to go to a restaurant or to the movies, but also make dates to go for walks or exercise. No matter what life throws at you, you can thrive, not just survive. If you are unhappy, tired, overweight, stressed, anxious, or depressed, exercise can act as an antidepressant. Exercise can help you heal, grow, and thrive. It will turn fear into faith. You don't have to run marathons, you just have to be more proactive about taking charge of your physical, emotional, and mental health.

Maybe you get excited about playing games on your mobile phone. That's fine, but also get excited about walking, workouts, swimming, yoga, biking, or playing a sport. Age well by engaging in adjusted physical activity. Your attitude determines the outcome of your health and illness. You have wellsprings of energy and health—tap into them. New beginnings make for great endings. It is never too late to make a change. Start small, start today. Life will then *not stop* after a major health crisis.

4

MOUNTAINEERING: MIND OVER BODY

You've got to win in your mind before you win in your life.

—JOHN ADDISON

Mount Kailash, Tibet (August 2010)

SOMETIME IN 2010, a friend asked me casually if I wanted to go trekking to Mount Kailash in Tibet. Without batting an eye, I said, "Sure."

After running my first half marathon, I was turning into an explorer and adventurer. If I came across anything daunting or challenging, I instantly agreed to be a part of it. My attitude and lifestyle had changed, and with newfound and unwavering energy and enthusiasm, I was ready to set goals that suited my newly acquired spirit of adventure.

Stretching my physical capabilities against all odds was now a distinct possibility because I had started to believe in the power of the mind and its potential to create cherished outcomes. "Let your mind take your body to places you never thought you would be able to," I would tell myself. "Don't belittle your mind. It will help uplift you to accomplish amazing feats that are beyond your wildest dreams."

Mount Kailash, hailed by Hindus as the abode of Lord Shiva, is a great mass of black rock with snow circling around. At its peak, it reaches 22,028 feet (6,714 meters), and is a deeply venerated site for Hindus, Buddhists, Jains, and Böns (indigenous religion of Tibet). Pilgrims from around the world go to this sacred mountain to circumambulate at about 19,000 feet, rather than scale the high peak. In fact, climbing Mount Kailash is forbidden. The only person to have ever climbed the holy mountain was Jetsun Milarepa, an eleventh-century Tibetan Buddhist yogi.

Devotees of Lord Shiva believe Shiva is eternal, omnipresent, and the supreme master of the universe. Within the Hindu trinity (this includes Lord Brahma and Vishnu), Shiva is considered the destroyer of evil. He is also known as Yogeshvara or the Lord of Yoga, who, although unmanifested, also exists in physical form atop the holy Kailash.

We started our overland trip in a bus from Kathmandu, Nepal. We crossed the Sino-Nepal Friendship Bridge to enter Tibet, covering a distance of 1,100 kilometers (683 miles) by road, from Kathmandu to the base camp of Mount Kailash.

Although this distance appears insignificant, we traversed some of the loftiest, steepest, and most uncomfortable terrains in the world, a fact that was confirmed by our tour guide, pilgrims who were on the bus with us, and our own experiences with the abysmal roads and precipitous slopes.

Once we entered Tibet, we were assigned into groups. Each group consisted of four people who would ride in a Toyota SUV to the base camp of Mount Kailash. But driving to the base was not easy. We encountered several landslides along the way, but apparently, this was commonplace. The roads were closed after each landslide, and we had to turn back to our previous location and wait for the road to be cleared before moving on.

We passed over narrow stretches, deep potholes, sheer cliffs, and rocks in a cloud of dust, the SUV bumping, stomping, twisting, and turning. I rode in sheer agony, my pain compounded by hemorrhoids. I was in a mess. It was a roller coaster ride for six or seven days.

At night, we stopped at whatever accommodations we could find.

The Nepalese company that had arranged our tour did not consider physical hardships and hygiene important factors in the undertaking of a *yatra* (pilgrimage). To them, since the pilgrims were high on devotion, they were fortified to adapt to any environment, even if it meant staying in squalid conditions. They called it adjusting while resting.

The first place we stopped, six to eight people had to share an unkempt and filthy room. My mattress was dusty, marked with stains, and had no bed cover. However, since we were all exhausted after our treacherous road journey, we didn't have the energy to resist or complain. All we wanted was sleep. But with so many people in one room, each one snoring louder than the other, it was not a very restful sleep. As if this weren't enough, we had to go outside to relieve ourselves since there were no indoor bathrooms.

Food that was given to us was limited, because in the tour company's mind, pilgrims are not foodies. Pilgrims consider food as prasāda (consecrated food), which is offered in small quantities to devotees. In the morning, we got around 120 mL of hot coffee in a tiny plastic cup, which felt as precious as gold. I have never savored coffee as much as I did on that trip.

The rejuvenating feature of the trip was the early morning prayers in the presence of the entire pilgrimage group. I participated in the prayers and bhajans (devotional songs). I wasn't a religious person, but the hymns and their melodious tones filled my mind and body with positive vibrations, solace, strength, and stillness … a feeling of being in unison with an unseen energy, inexplicable in words.

Pilgrimages are never meant to be easy. You are not on a holiday. They are arduous and uncomfortable, and are meant to test us. The drive was overwhelming and tiring, the food was limited, the living conditions pathetic, but all that taught me a great lesson—acceptance. That which can't be changed must be endured with acceptance.

During the journey, we had to drink a lot of water and were on diuretics for altitude sickness. It was getting colder, and oxygen was getting scarcer. It was difficult, but nothing that I couldn't withstand.

Through the harsh terrain with lots of ups and downs, we seemed to march forever till we reached one of the most beautiful lakes in the world, Lake Manasarovar, the world's highest freshwater lake. The snow-covered mountains of the Kailash range were reflected in the waters of the lake, and were in splendid and majestic contrast with the deep turquoise-blue colors of the lake.

The pristine and holy water of Lake Manasarovar was beckoning us to take a plunge. It is believed that taking a dip in the icy water washes away negative or bad karmas. I didn't get into the lake to purify myself. I took the plunge because I felt a magnetic pull and was drawn in by its grandeur.

The water was awfully cold. But once I got into the lake, it didn't bother me. The transcendent moments of pure joy and exhilaration that I experienced overpowered the teeth-chattering joy of freezing cold water. A wave of calmness and peace washed over me that I had never experienced before. I was one with nature, healed, refreshed, and uplifted.

After the blissful pause at the venerated Lake Manasarovar, it was time to continue our journey and get to Darchen, the village at the southern foot of Mount Kailash.

We had embarked on our expedition at Kathmandu and journeyed onward on a trying route that encompassed Dram, Nyalam, Saga, Paryang, and Lake Manasarovar. We were still miles away from Darchen, which stands at an elevation of 15,338 feet (4,675 meters), the starting point for the actual pilgrimage to the revered Mount Kailash.

Thankfully, we arrived in one piece at Darchen. The skilled drivers had brought us this far and couldn't go any farther. From here on, we had to undertake the yatra on foot, a pony, or yak. The three-day Mount Kailash pilgrimage begins at Darchen, but before that, I had to make the major decision whether to continue onward on foot or use a pony to take me up the mountain.

Out of the group of thirty people, only four of us decided to do the entire three-day pilgrimage on foot. This included my friend and I, and two women from London who were younger (presumably in their forties) but who had never ever done even a 2K run. I call this divine faith, which not only moves mountains, but also makes you walk mountains.

At an altitude of over 15,000 feet, I was quite literally on top of the world. I had not felt this good, emotionally and physically, since the completion of my first half marathon in Nashville, Tennessee.

The three-day pilgrimage, which involves walking around the thirty-two-mile (fifty-two- kilometer) circumference of Mount Kailash, is referred to as *parikrama* by Hindus, Buddhists, and Jains, and as the *Kora* by Böns. The Hindus, Buddhist, and Jains do the parikrama clockwise while the Böns do it counterclockwise.

The expedition from Darchen took us to Dolma La Pass at 18,471 feet (5,560 meters). This was the highest permissible point for pilgrims to ascend. No one is allowed to go up any farther due to Mount Kailash's sacred status.

On the first day of our three-day journey, we worked our way up Chaktsal Gang to Drirapuk Gompa (17,093 feet or 5,210 meters). The second day was the toughest part of the pilgrimage, as we had to continue trekking uphill to the highest pass, Dolma La Pass (5,560 meters or 18,471 feet), where a big boulder that represents the Goddess Dolma (Dolma La is the Tibetan name of Goddess Parvati, wife of Lord Shiva) is festooned with prayer flags. The Dolma La Pass is the highest physical and spiritual point of the parikrama or kora.

People have died here. I didn't know this then.

According to the Singaporean newspaper *The New Paper*, in 2012, two Singaporeans died after developing altitude sickness at the Dolma La Pass.

In June 2016, *Hindustan Times*, a prominent English-language daily newspaper in India, reported that three Indians and one Canadian of Indian origin died from altitude sickness (their ages ranged from fifty-nine to seventy-six years) while undertaking the Kailash Manasarovar Yatra.

At one stage, the officials insisted I get a yak or a pony. They also asked to see my cardiac clearance. I candidly admitted that I'd had a bypass surgery a year or so ago, but now I was in great physical condition and could comfortably complete the circumambulation on foot. I had to use all my persuasion skills, including the fact that I was a doctor. They begrudgingly agreed.

During the formidable three-day peregrination, the one constant was continual walking. We stopped only for tea, coffee or lunch, or camping for the night in a tent. It was freezing cold, and there were no showers or restrooms. In fact, we couldn't shower or change our clothes during the seventy-two-hour expedition. We were extremely uncomfortable, having to wear the same clothes and lacking basic facilities during the entire excursion, particularly because of adverse weather conditions. Yet we persevered, our intense drive and determination helping us stay motivated and focused to complete the parikrama.

Once we got to the Dolma La Pass, emotions got the best of me. I was teary-eyed and overjoyed all at once. Fellow yatris were congratulating each other, but I craved isolation. I needed space, which made the people around me uncomfortable. I sat on a rock away from the crowd, and felt for the first time what life would be like if you were devoid of material comforts and luxuries and yet had this immense inner peace that can only be felt, seldom described.

As expected, we took longer to go up than come down from the mountain, but the adventure was far from over. On our way down, we encountered hail; and as if this weren't enough, we had to spend the night in tents that were flooded due to fierce thunderstorms. The heavy downpour of rain continued for six or seven hours. My enlarged prostate caused me anguish, and I had to step out of the tent amidst the torrential rains to relieve myself.

After our descent and return to Darchen, we were desperate to shower and get into a fresh clothes. While walking around Darchen, we found a small store that let us use the hot shower for a fee and that lasted only about eight minutes. They gave each of us a towel and a small bar of soap. I took off my clothes as quickly as I could because the time had started as soon as I handed the money. I was freezing till I got in the shower. Oh, what a feeling. I did not have to use the soap. The grime and dirt that washed down my body was like a layer of skin coming off. It was indeed the best shower I'd ever had.

I still get goosebumps thinking about circumambulating Mount Kailash, particularly completing the parikrama route at an elevation of 18,500 feet on foot. There were times when I badly wanted to give up, but my faith in my abilities to overcome insurmountable challenges saw me through.

The journey that started and ended in Kathmandu, Nepal, took two weeks to complete. The trip to Mount Kailash was a challenging yet profound journey, and the arduous expedition had transformed me. Not only did I learn the meaning of acceptance, but also the importance of spending quality time with myself. Mount Kailash reminded me how blessed I am, and reinforced my belief that with conviction, humility, faith, and fearlessness, we can make it through the trying but joyous terrain that is life.

When you go to Mount Kailash, you go on a journey that is both inward and outward. All the hardships I had gone through seemed trivial once I returned home. Upon my return, people noticed I had become a calmer version of myself.

I experienced unusual spiritual occurrences that I could not grasp through intellectual reasoning, but I knew they felt right. My definition of spirituality helped me from then on to live in the moment in peace and to handle problems better.

I can now be alone yet not feel lonely. It has taken me decades to get to this state of mind. I enjoy my own company more than I did ever before, perhaps because I have become more contemplative and observant.

Mount Kailash added another adventurous twist to my exciting new life, and helped me understand the power of the mind. I told my family and friends, "I have learned to strengthen my mind, and that's helped take me further in the last year than most people go in decades. I have no regrets. However, I wish I had the mind I have now in the youthful body I had then."

Mount Kilimanjaro, Tanzania (September 2012) The World's Tallest Free-Standing Mountain

Challenges make you discover things about yourself that you never really knew.

—CICELY TYSON

A journey up is a journey within.

After Mount Kailash in Tibet, I climbed Pike's Peak in Colorado (14,000 feet or 4,267.2 meters) and Le Conte Peak in the Great Smoky

Mountains National Park, which rises to 6,593 feet (2,010 meters). All three mountains were a prelude to my climbing Mount Kilimanjaro in 2012, the highest point on the African continent. In a sense, the experiences I had during the preparation and climbing of the first three mountains were greatly useful, not only in building my stamina and strength, but also in building my mental state. In retrospect, however, Mount Kilimanjaro proved to be something far beyond my expectations, even knowing it is the highest free-standing mountain in the world and the fourth highest of the coveted Seven Summits of the world, of which Mount Everest is the highest.

Kilimanjaro lies 205 miles (330 kilometers) south of the equator in the country of Tanzania. Kilimanjaro once had three volcanic cones: Kibo, Shira, and Mawenzi. Kibo is the tallest cone, and that's where the summit stands. Shira has collapsed, creating the Shira Plateau on the western side of the mountain. Mawenzi is a craggy peak standing 5,149 meters (16,896 feet) tall, and is the third highest peak in Africa, after Kibo and Mount Kenya. Shira and Mawenzi are extinct volcanoes. However, Kibo is a dormant volcano; it can erupt again. The last major eruption was 360,000 years ago. The most recent activity was 200,000 years ago.[2]

I started training four months prior to the climb. Besides the training, I had to make sure I purchased the right gear and took the required shots, including the mandatory shots for yellow fever.

My sister, Fatima, had died a few months before my climb. She and I had shared a deep bond. I was saddened by this untimely loss, but continued with my plans as she would have wanted. She was one of my ardent supporters, and I decided to dedicate this climb to her.

I arrived at the Kilimanjaro International Airport, the closest airport to the small town of Moshi, which is the capital of the Kilimanjaro region in northeastern Tanzania and situated on the lower slopes of the scenic mountain. From the airport, my friend, his wife and daughter, and I drove nearly nineteen miles to get to Moshi. Nafisa planned to fly to Tanzania in a week, to join me for a wildlife safari after the climb.

The Keys Hotel in Moshi offered us an incredible view of Mount Kilimanjaro. I stood there enchanted, feasting on the majestic splendor of the mountain. Suffice to say that no photo can ever do justice to what I saw. Several other tour groups were there for the climb and were using shorter routes, the Marangu (Coca-Cola) Route and the Machame (Whiskey) Route, but we had chosen the scenic eight-day Lemosho Route. The Marangu Route is considered touristy and offers sleeping huts that serve beverages like Coca-Cola on the way. The Machame Route is tougher, and hence is sometimes called the whiskey route. One reason for using the longer route was to help with acclimatization. There were six in our group: two women in their twenties, my friend in his early fifties, his wife in her forties, and a pulmonologist and I, both of us in our sixties. That night, I couldn't sleep much. Maybe it was the excitement of the start of the climb the next day.

Early in the morning, after breakfast, an experienced guide gave us a pre-climb briefing.

The most important advice was *pole pole* (pronounced po-lay, po-lay in Swahili), which means *slowly, slowly*. The point of pole pole was that one must walk slowly up the mountain to keep the heart rate low (so as not to lose too much oxygen), and to help the body acclimatize as you gain elevation. One must never rush or walk fast. By the same token, one can never walk too slow. The slow walk became a mantra for us as we climbed the mountain, and I often heard fellow climbers reciting, "Pole pole."

The mountaineer's old maxim is to climb higher and rest/sleep lower to acclimatize the body to the altitude and avoid mountain sickness. This meant that when we got to the camping site in the late afternoon or early evening, we walked a few thousand feet on and then returned to the campsite.

In December 2010, tennis legend Martina Navratilova was forced to abandon her climb on Mount Kilimanjaro after she had trouble breathing, and she had to be hospitalized for pulmonary edema (fluid in the lungs). This served as a warning to me. Altitude knows no body type and does not care how awesome you are. Altitude sickness, the symptoms of which are exhaustion, shortness of breath, headache, and trouble focusing, also took its toll on the pulmonologist in our group. He finished the climb, but he was later diagnosed with pulmonary edema in the

United States and was hospitalized for a few days. Luckily, he recovered completely.

Malaria was also a problem in Tanzania. A good thing for us climbers was that the risk of contracting malaria was inversely proportional to the altitude we attained. We were highly unlikely to be affected once we climbed above 6,000 feet (1,828.8 meters) because the mosquitoes that carry the malarial parasite do not survive at higher altitudes. However, we did take Malarone (an antimalarial drug) when we were in Moshi, the altitude of which was less than 6,000 feet (1,828.8 meters). Little did I know then that in a few hours, a side effect of Malarone would lead me to nearly abandon the climb. We also took Diamox two days before the climb for altitude sickness, and, as advised by the guides, drank four to five liters of water per day.

There were, of course, no shower facilities during the climb, but we all had to poop and pee. For doing our business (sending a short or a long message, as they called it on the mountain) we used portable toilets, nifty little devices that come with their own tents and are carried by porters from one campsite to another. Toilets are a topic that never really gets mentioned in day-to-day life. However, on Kilimanjaro a person's toilet adventures become a hot topic of conversation. During the climb, if we had to relieve ourselves (long message), we went to the bushes, dug a hole with a little spade we carried, did our business, and covered the hole with mud. We cleaned ourselves with wet wipes, which we carried in ziplock bags to be disposed at the next campsite. Don't you hate it when nature calls on you when you are in nature!

We were fortunate that besides the experienced mountain guides who assisted us during the climb, the porters carried the camping equipment and cooks prepared meals for us. Food was good and plentiful. Breakfast consisted of porridge, eggs, toast, honey, and fresh fruit. Lunch was usually a short break from the trek, but we had pasta salads, pies, fajitas, and hardboiled eggs. Dinner was delicious, with vegetable soups, potato salad, jerk chicken, vegetable and potato stew, apple pancakes, and crepes for dessert. As for me, there were enough vegetarian items to see me through. Even though the same food was served to us throughout the ascent, it was so good that we all looked forward to it after our day's climb.

The Lemosho Route approaches Mount Kilimanjaro from the west, beginning with a four-hour drive from Moshi to Londorossi Gate, where we completed our registration formalities and met our mountain guides. We then drove for another hour on a muddy and slippery road to the Lemosho trailhead. Here we commenced trekking through the undisturbed and untouched rainforest.

We traversed a distance of four miles to reach Mt. Mkubwa Camp (at 8,695 feet or 2,650 meters), where we camped for the night. The trek to the camp took us four hours to complete as we religiously adhered to pole pole. Time and time again, our patience to take small steps was tested in covering such a short distance in such a long time, but none of us were foolish enough to hurry.

I had expected the first day to be a climb of one or two miles, but we continued up the mountain to an altitude of 1,795 feet (547.116 meters). While the climb was hard physically, each one of us was rejuvenated by the stimulation of our visual sense—the myriad changes in topography as we climbed through the thick and dark rainforest to open grounds that displayed colorful flowers. It was a sight I am sure even *National Geographic* photos would struggle to compete with. Even the shy and harmless colobus and blue monkeys lent beauty to the area with their presence.

Our camp for the night was close to 9,000 feet (2,743.2 meters), and given that darkness comes early in the forest, we had only an hour before dinner to rest our fatigued bodies and prepare for the next morning. We ate well and drank at least a liter of water before going to bed. We all needed to build up energy reserves for the higher altitudes, where there is an increased possibility of losing one's appetite.

As I tried to put my tired body to sleep, I couldn't. The side effects of the antimalarial medication were beginning to show up as insomnia and anxiety. I stayed awake all night. At first, I talked to my friend next to me, till he and the guys in the other tents asked me to shut up. With my enlarged prostate, all the fluids I'd drunk, and the water pills I'd taken, I kept getting a strong urge to pee every two to three hours. It was frigid outside, so I fumbled around in the pitch dark, trying to find my headlamp so I could find my pee bottle. I then rolled onto my side, still in my sleeping bag, made the necessary adjustments, and waited anxiously for the flow. Nothing happened. Frustrated, I got onto my knees. My friend asked what I was doing.

I meekly answered, "Praying for a miracle." And finally it happened, and oh, my God, what a relief!

I wondered if my one liter bottle would hold the two or three liters of water I had drunk during the day. I had to get up several times during the night, and finally my pee bottle was full. I had only two choices now. Hold it till the next morning, or go out in the frigid cold. I went out.

The next morning around eight, after breakfast, we continued on the trail, which lead out of the rainforest and into a savannah of tall grasses, where heather and volcanic rocks were draped with lacy, greenish lichen beards. Our schedule called for a full day trek of five miles, climbing 3,650 feet (960 meters), that would take us between five to six hours.

The trail was very steep, and we took more breaks than we had the previous day. After trekking slowly for almost half the distance, we stopped for lunch just outside the scenic Shira Crater at around 9,845 feet (3,000 meters). By now, we had left the forest behind and entered the moorland zone with its giant heathers, as we worked our way up toward the Shira Plateau. A well-deserved lunch break helped me catch a breath and rest my tired legs and mildly puffy feet.

After lunch, we climbed through the rolling hills, one ridge after another, hiking higher and higher to reach the Shira Ridge, a high-altitude desert plateau, before descending gently down to Shira 1 Camp at 11,500 feet (3,505.2 meters). Shira Plateau is the third of Kilimanjaro's volcanic cones, and is filled with lava flow from the Kibo Peak. We caught our first glimpse of the majestic Kibo across the plateau. It was an exquisite view, with diverse plants, rock formations, and several streams. We reached Shira Camp around 4:30 to rest for the night. Later in the evening, we experienced sleet.

That night, I was once again struck by insomnia. I had had tremendous energy all day that had helped me make it to Shira 1 Camp, even though sleep had escaped me the past night. Yet, staying up all night was making me restless and moody. The thought of not getting any sleep was worse than not getting any sleep. I knew fatigue would catch up with me sooner or later. The prospect of not being able to sleep hit me so hard, for a moment I thought of abandoning the climb.

Fortunately, there were certain spots where I got a cell phone signal, so I was able to call my wife and tell her about my plans. Her warm and caring words kept me going well until the early hours of the morning. They eased my irritable disposition and nervousness into positive energy and enthusiasm.

Witnessing the breathtaking view of the sun rising behind Kibo the next morning finally calmed me, filling me with resilience. I felt invigorated, raring to face the exhausting day that awaited us. Our first goal for the day was to get to Lava Tower (15,190 feet), a 300-foot volcanic rock formation left over from when Kilimanjaro was volcanic. From Shira, we were to journey on to the east toward Kibo, passing the junction with the circular route and then onward toward the Lava Tower.

The day started with a brief but steep climb. Due to the altitude gain, some of our group felt short of breath and listless. One of them had an asthma attack, while my colleague, the pulmonologist, was having a hard time breathing. But their spirits were high, and when supplemental oxygen (O2) was provided, they got better. I too was getting a bit short of breath, and my legs were getting heavier due to lactic acid buildup. The important thing was to get sufficient O2 to keep functioning while using as little energy as possible. The trick was to take a step, inhale, rest, and exhale. Even if you are resting on a rock, you never, ever rest your deep breathing. Step, inhale, rest, and exhale became a mantra to me. It also had to be done very slowly. It was like watching yourself in slow motion.

The well-trained guides helped us deal with altitude sickness (AS). Twice a day, they gave us a medical checkup, monitoring our vital signs, listening to our lung sounds, doing the pulse oximetry, which measures the O2 saturation in the blood. Normal O2 saturation levels are between 95 and 100 percent. Anything below 95 percent is low, and supplemental O2 was given if the need arose. They also saw to it that we were well hydrated and asked about our bowel movements. We saw a climber from another group being taken down in a wheelbarrow because he was dehydrated, secondary to severe diarrhea. They also inquired about any other problems we might be having, and if we were sleeping well.

Looking toward Kibo, we could see the trail ahead crossing several ridges and valleys. As we continued our march, we gradually left the heather and moorland behind and entered the mostly barren alpine desert region, where the rocky landscapes resembled the surface of the moon. These are uncongenial frigid conditions where plant life is largely reduced to mosses and lichens.

Our long hike, with pathways that took us up and down, some with ninety-degree turns, continued until our trail converged with the Machame Route. This trek was exhausting, but my fatigue gave way to a sigh of relief when we descended all the way down to the Lava Tower. We had climbed up to over 15,000 feet (4,572 meters), and I could hear the sound of my own labored breathing.

After lunch near the Lava Tower, we descended to Barranco Camp at an altitude of 13,000 feet (3,962.4 meters). It was one of the most beautiful campsites of the Lemosho Route, with heart-stirring views of Kibo, the Western Breach (considered the most technically challenging route to Kilimanjaro), and the beginning of the southern glaciers.

Although we began the day at 12,467 feet (3,800 meters) and ended at approximately the same elevation—12,795 feet (3,900 meters)—the time spent at a higher altitude (4,500 meters) proved to be beneficial for acclimatization and avoiding altitude sickness.

We paused for the night. The temperature had dipped. It was cold and frosty. Knowing I couldn't continue the hike without sleep, and fearing I would have problems sleeping again, I had thrown caution to the winds and not taken the antimalarial medication. That night, I slept peacefully.

The next morning, our objective was a short but steep hike that would likely appear a lot longer than the three miles we were to cover that day. We had breakfast a little later than normal and departed for our next stop to Karanga Valley at 10:00.

We descended into a ravine to the base of the Barranco Wall, a steep, nearly 900 feet (274.32 meters) cliff, climbing over rock, gravel, and loose stones. We slowed our pace considerably in climbing the wall, taking care not to twist our ankles. There were times when we had to crawl and use all four limbs to scramble up the wall, and to lunge from one large rock to another. I was thankful I'd practiced lunges during my training back home. Some parts of the path were very narrow, especially the patch around the Kissing Rock, where the guides helped us. One wrong move, and it was straight down in the valley.

When we crossed the last section to the wall, we were greeted by cheers, hugs, and high fives from the people who had already made it. From the top of the wall, we crossed a series of hills and valleys until the trail descended sharply into Karanga Valley. From there, we had a steeper climb out of the valley to the Karanga Camp. In spite of the short distance of three miles, it took us almost five hours to get there. We lunched at Karanga Camp and remained there for the night.

Our next uphill sojourn to Barafu Camp was barely two miles in length but would take us five hours. Barafu Camp, at an altitude of 15,331 feet (4,672.88 meters), was our penultimate destination in the Kilimanjaro voyage. We left Karanga Valley and hit the junction that connected with the Mweka Trail, trudging up the rocky section of the trail to Barafu Camp. The air up here was cold and thin, lacking much oxygen. Under these conditions and at that height, helicopter evacuation was not possible. We felt truly isolated, knowing there was no easy way out for us if something were to happen. Once again, a few from our group had to use O2. Our guides made sure we adhered to the pole pole credo as we made our way across jagged rock and slate, layered with a loose layer of soil. We reached Barafu Camp in the afternoon. We were exhausted, and the altitude and cold were getting on to us. It even made getting across camp difficult.

At this point, we had completed the Southern Circuit, which had offered us spectacular panoramic views. We were merely eight hours away from the most daunting challenge on this trek: climbing Uhuru Peak, 19,341 feet (5,894.832 meters), the highest point on Mount Kilimanjaro.

After dinner, we went to bed early that night. Our ascent was going to begin at four in the morning. Most of us got little sleep. It was more resting than sleeping, wondering what was in store for us the next day. Some climbers ascend at midnight to catch the sunrise at Uhuru Peak. A few in our group preferred to rest more and start in the morning. At around 4:00 a.m., we enjoyed hot coffee and breakfast, and then started our climb to the summit. It was dark. It was cold and windy. For a while, we could not see anything except the headlamps of those ahead of us.

This was going to be the most mentally, emotionally, and physically grueling and exhausting portion of the trek. Our first major goal was to hike to Stella Point, just a shade under 19,000 feet.

We walked in the dark over frozen ground for a couple hours, till the first rays of the sun hit us. Sunrise was pretty awesome, and I wanted to take a picture but did not have the strength to do so. We had to take frequent, short breaks. We were now going at a snail's pace.

Pole pole!

I listened to my labored breathing, and the dry air hurt my throat as I tried to take in as much O_2 as I could with each breath. I watched my legs wobble as if I were carrying a huge weight.

I started my mantra. Step, inhale, rest, exhale. Slowly, we marched up, planting our trekking poles, shuffling along. My feet kept moving as if detached from me, but I knew I would make it as long as I kept moving.

Our group had broken up. The pulmonologist and my friend's wife needed extra help, so they were assigned a guide each. They were both on O2. The two young women were way ahead and had a guide to themselves. So, my friend and I had to settle with one porter and no guide. We rested along the scree switchbacks that lead to Stella Point to have a picnic lunch of the sandwiches we had carried with us.

After six hours of ascending the steep section, we made it to Stella Point. Stella Point is at the edge of Crater Rim. Climbers who reach the Point receive the official Kilimanjaro climbing certificate and can deservedly claim they reached the top of Kilimanjaro. But I had not come this far not to climb Uhuru Peak.

The spectacular views along this journey and my penchant for thrill and adventure, backed by faith, perseverance, and a dogged determination to surmount all obstacles, helped me march onward to Uhuru Peak, the mother of all excruciatingly strenuous hikes on Kilimanjaro and situated a mere two hours away. Or so we were told. We walked along the wide paths of the crater rim that allowed glimpses down onto massive glaciers shining in the afternoon sun. The climb to Uhuru Peak was merely a mile in distance, but it wasn't two hours of hiking as we were led to believe. It was a lot more.

It was the ultimate test of endurance, facing unimaginable, bone-chilling cold and high altitude (over 19,000 feet); and low oxygen saturation, which meant that with every breath, less oxygen was being delivered to our muscles and brain. The bitter cold and low oxygen conditions made us appear as aging, slow-moving tortoises gasping for air, caught between desperately trying to inhale enough oxygen when we felt like we were almost out of breath and the tenacious persistence that drove us ever closer to the coveted Uhuru Peak.

I wore layers of warm clothes that included fleeces, a waterproof jacket, a down jacket, trekking trousers (fleece lined and waterproof), mittens, thermal socks, a balaclava knit cap that covered my head, neck, and the top of my shoulders, and a wooly hat on top of the knit cap. For the lower part of my legs, I wore resilient trekking boots that covered my lower legs. But, in spite of my careful adherence to my clothing and trekking gear, the last phase of the five-hour hike—the last mile—from Stella Point to Uhuru Peak was, perhaps, the hardest part of the climb. My body started to crumble, and I had to take a short break about every hundred feet. As time dragged on, I felt I was not moving. I was so exhausted that I began falling asleep standing up, my trekking poles keeping me upright. The summit I'd thought was so close kept getting farther and farther away. But sheer willpower ruled the day, and I reached Uhuru Peak, the highest point in Africa, standing majestically tall at a height of 19,341 feet.

I was elevated, triumphant even, to have reached the top. To para-phrase Julius Caesar, "I came, I saw, I conquered." But it was far from the truth. I was humbled by the grandness of the mountaineering excursion.

My eyes filled with tears of overwhelming happiness and relief. I had completed the journey of a lifetime, with a new but *open heart*. The discomfort born from prolonged exposure to extreme cold, the struggle with breathing, and the exhaustion from the arduous climb waned in comparison to the euphoria we experienced having made it to the top of Mount Kilimanjaro.

We stayed at the summit for about fifteen minutes to soak in the moment and take a few pictures. Suddenly, I remembered that I had carried my grandson's pacifier and a sliver of my trainer's wedding dress, as she had asked me to, to leave at the peak. They were both with me, but I could not find them. Finally, I gave up. Later on, at the base camp, I did locate both, and they are still with me to this day as mementos of my climb. I did thank my old heart too. Had it not led me onto the path of bypass surgery, the indolent physician would only have had mundane memories of an unexciting, purposeless life.

I now had a newfound respect for Mother Nature. This is where the art and science of a fulfilling life converge. While climbing Kilimanjaro, we had hiked through gale-force winds and snow, and five distinct ecological zones ranging from tropical to arid, rain to arctic.

Each zone got colder—my fingers got frosted at times—and drier as the elevation increased. At the peak, the weather was in the arctic zone, and there was no plant or animal life because of the lack of oxygen and intense cold. The temperature ranged from 0 to -5 degrees Fahrenheit, and the oxygen level was less than half of what is found at sea level. And not to forget the unbuffered and powerful sun that required us to wear sunglasses to protect us from sun blindness and sun-induced headaches caused by the sun's direct brilliance and its reflection off the ice-covered ground. A porter accompanying us suffered the pain of continual sun-caused headaches. It was one more reason why our guides performed medical checks on us twice a day.

Still, we had reached the top, a desolate place of ice and rock where nothing grew and the air barely contained any oxygen. Amidst these treacherous conditions, we remained steadfast, clinging to our inner strength, carefully progressing farther, moving pole pole. The entire experience of climbing to the top was humbling, though. It made me realize that we humans are a mere speck in the creation of Mother Nature.

But the expedition was not over yet!

After taking the celebratory photos, we began our steep but picturesque descent, continuing straight down to the Mweka Camp, stopping at Barafu Camp for lunch. Descending from 19,341 feet to 10,065 feet sounded like a lot of fun, but it was not. It was hard on the knees because of the downward slope, and the rocks, sand, and scree. On our ascent, we had zigzagged back and forth to reduce the uphill grade, but on the descent, we took the slope straight on. It was all downhill in pitch dark except for my porter's and my headlamps. The guides were still with people who needed help in our group. My friend, who had been with me on the way up, had slowed down considerably, helping his wife. I found myself stopping less often and just pushing on through the pain and exhaustion. Every so often, I would slip on the scree and lose my balance. We hardly took any breaks, and it was getting extremely windy and cold. Finally, we reached the sandy part of the trail where I could take larger steps, but with each step, my foot hit sand and slid a few feet till I could plant my other foot. It felt like I was skiing down, using my trekking poles for balance.

While descending, I noticed that Kilimanjaro's glaciers are shrinking and thinning. According to Pascal Sirguey, a research scientist at the University of Otago in New Zealand, Kilimanjaro's shrinking northern glaciers, thought to be 10,000 years old, could disappear by 2030. This was the first time I realized the devastating effects of global warming. I had seen pictures of what Kilimanjaro looked like ten years ago, and that was in sharp contrast to what I witnessed while trekking downhill. I now understood what Wallace Smith Broecker, the longtime Columbia University professor and renowned climate scientist who popularized the term *global warming*, meant when he said, "The climate system is an angry beast and we are poking it with sticks."

Finally, after a seven-mile hike, we reached Mweka Camp in the late afternoon. I went straight to my tent, got into my sleeping bag, and instantly fell asleep. Later in the evening, we celebrated our climb, relating our adventure with nostalgia, joy, and a feeling of fulfillment. We sang, danced, bantered, and joked. Our trekking group had plenty of stories and experiences to share. It was our last night on Mount Kilimanjaro, and we enjoyed our last dinner and a well-earned sleep.

The next morning, we continued a four-hour descent through the pretty rainforest to Mweka Gate, where we collected our badge of honor, the summit certificate. Sadly, it was time to say good-bye to our team of experienced mountain guides, porters, and cooks. The last day of the journey ended with an hour's walk to Mweka Village. From the village, we were driven back to Keys Hotel in Moshi.

The hike to Mount Kilimanjaro heightened my self-awareness. It made me realize my true physical and emotional capabilities, and the extent to which I could push my established limits. I could go so far only because I let my mind take my body to places I never thought I would be able to conquer.

Unlike marathons, which end after some intense hours of running, this climb ended after a grueling eight-day hike in the face of extreme weather conditions, oxygen-deprived breathing, and steep ascents and descents. As someone in my group said, it is challenging the first time, but you have to be a fool to repeat it.

At Moshi, I was greeted by Nafisa. She had come a day earlier to wait for me. She could not believe what she saw. My hair was matted and shaggy, my nail beds were bleeding with small pockets of pus at several places. I had no idea that my backpack smelled of urine, even though I had washed the pee pot every chance I got. But she was relieved to see me in one piece.

Before we could celebrate my successful climb, a shower was a far more pressing need. I hadn't showered for eight days, and I needed to take a warm one immediately before I forgot what being clean felt like.

The next day, Nafisa and I were off to Ngorongoro Crater Safari, also the home of the Masai tribe. We had arranged this with Tusker Trail, the American outfitters my group had used for our climb. To be honest, I remember little of the safari, as most of the time I remained a zombie or asleep. The only animals that I recall are zebras and wildebeest. However, according to Nafisa, the other members of the safari group saw four of the Big Five—lion, elephant, buffalo, and rhino. In retrospect, I wish I had done the safari prior to the climb.

Go forth and strengthen your mind

We belittle our minds, but if you give it a chance, you'll see it's amazing. A powerful and positive mindset has the potential to create cherished or evolved outcomes.

My philosophy:

Have immense faith in yourself and in a higher power.
Train, persist, and stay dedicated.
Remind yourself to constantly keep mind over matter.
Remember that adventure may hurt you, but monotony will kill you.

5

EMBRACE THE FUN, THE
FALL, AND THE UNKNOWN

*My attitude has always been, if you fall flat on your face, at least
you're moving forward. All you have to do is get back up and
try again.*

—RICHARD BRANSON

Triathlon, Mud Race, and 100-Mile Biking

IT WAS 2013, a time when I craved excitement, doing anything that had a sense of adventure with a hint of a challenge. In this context, it occurred to me I had not run the triathlon, a multisport race that includes swimming, biking, and running.

Besides being a challenging event, the triathlon seemed to be a fun event, and I undertook it in the company of two of my nephews, a neighbor, and a late friend's daughter. We decided on the Lake Lanier, Georgia, triathlon, which starts with a quarter-mile shoreline swim, followed by a thirteen-mile bike ride, and a three-mile run.

Marathons in the past had tested my running skills, and I was quite sure a mere three-mile run would be a cinch for me. My biggest doubt about completing the race was the bike portion. I had always felt bicycling was not for me, even though I had no real rationale to justify my uneasiness in riding a bike. It was not that I didn't know how to ride a bike, which I occasionally did as a family activity. But during such times, I seldom had any concerns about the type of bicycle I was riding. For competitive speed biking, I would have to master riding a lightweight racing bike with skinny tires that required constant gear changing to accommodate different inclines, up and down.

First, I had to learn how to mount the bike. My idea of mounting a bike was to put one foot on a pedal and push the bike forward with the other foot, then cross the leg over onto the other side, similar to mounting a horse. With my racing bike, I now stood astride the bike in front of the seat, one foot on the ground and the other on the pedal, which allowed me to roll forward and pull myself up on the seat. I had to do this with clip-less pedals, where shoes are held in place by a spring mechanism (cleats) that locks the feet to the pedals. This allows the feet to stay in a consistent position, and the biker can use power more efficiently.

It's true that for people new to clipping, a *zero–speed* fall is inevitable. This happens when you stop moving forward but don't allow enough time to unhinge your foot from the pedal. After several falls and a few bruises, I became an expert at falling. The biggest bruise was to my ego. I also had to learn how to shift gears effectively and how to brake correctly, especially before stopping or slowing down in a group. But there were other things, such as learning to pedal smoothly and manage a climb based on my size and height. More importantly, I learned how to stay within my limits while creating new limits. Learning to ride a bicycle as a competitive sport certainly wasn't as easy as I had expected.

With the help of my nephew Munir and my friend Naresh, I began to appreciate the correct method for riding a sports bicycle. Within a few months, I got so comfortable with riding my bike, I saw it more as an extension of myself than a separate vehicle that would get me from one place to another. I biked thrice a week, each time spending over an hour on my bike. It was not long before I became a part of the biking culture, discussing its lexicon with the others in our group.

But the greatest challenge I faced for the triathlon was swimming, a challenge that was partly my own making. Swimming just a quarter mile seemed within my reach, even though I never prided myself on my swimming skills. I could only do the breaststroke, which is the slowest of the four competitive strokes. Most triathletes do the freestyle, which is a lot faster.

To face the cold waters of Lake Lanier, I decided to buy a full-body wet suit online. In my excitement, I immediately put it on when it arrived without reading the instructions, which specifically required me to apply body glide on my wrists, legs, toes, ankles, feet, and all around my neck to help get the suit on and off with ease. As it was, it took me a while to get it on, but I could not take it off, no matter how hard I tried.

I sat on the bed, took a few deep breaths for a final effort to get it off, and managed to pull the wet suit down to my waist. But that was it. I could not get it off the lower part of my body. I tried as hard as I could before swallowing my pride and leaving the room to get help.

I came down to my living room and asked my bemused wife for help. She took hold of both rubber leggings and tried to drag me out of it, but it didn't work.

Eventually, Nafisa got a pair of scissors and cut about five inches on the outer side of each legging. She now had a better grip to not only pull the wet suit off me, but also a whole lot of hair off my legs. We laughed our lungs out as we created a spontaneous moment of togetherness in a most unexpected manner.

Since I had never swum with a wet suit, I decided to get used to it at the local YMCA swimming pool. This time, I made sure to use body glide before putting on the suit.

It felt great to have the protective covering of the wet suit against the cold, but I immediately realized I could not move while doing the breaststroke. Try as hard as I could, all I did was float on the surface like a balloon. No article, journal, or book mentioned that one cannot do the breaststroke wearing a wet suit, and I had no way of knowing from other swimmers in my group because they seldom used the breaststroke.

And so, the cold water conundrum continued.

I couldn't make myself plunge into the cold water. I tried to find other methods online, but there were no external devices that could help me with my dilemma. A part of me wanted to give up, but since I was a firm believer in being in harmony with what nature provided, that was not an option for me.

Eventually, I decided to take the bull by its horns and face the cold water by gradually acclimatizing myself to the environment I would have to face. For a week before the triathlon, I took a cold-water shower every morning. I then poured a bucket of ice-cold water over myself that had my teeth chattering. I did this ritually every day for seven days. By the day of the triathlon, I had become used to the cold water.

On September 29, 2013, we started at the Lake Lanier Island Triathlon near Atlanta, Georgia. I swam the cold waters of Lake Lanier, biked thirteen miles, and completed the three-mile run. It felt great to complete the course, standing second in my age group that year.

Learning how to fall, embracing ice-cold water, being dragged like a rag doll to try to get out of a stuck wet suit … all happening at sixty-four.

But for me, at the age of sixty-four, having fun was a continuing process. I was already wondering about my next adventure.

Udder Mud Run—Obstacle Course Racing (August 2015)

The only thing that makes life possible is permanent, intolerable uncertainty; not knowing what comes next.

—URSULA K. LE GUIN

My next quest was to run the 2015 Udder Mud Run. The mud run was held at the Future Farmers of America—Family, Career and Community Leaders of America (FFA-FCCLA) Georgia Center in Covington, Georgia.

The FFA-FCCLA mud run, also known as Obstacle Course Racing (OCR), is a 7K (4 miles) muddy course with various types of obstacles on a challenging terrain. It has been increasing in popularity over the years. Nearly 1,200 people participated in the run in 2015. Just as my daughter had joined me to run the Mumbai marathon, my son, Nikhil, decided to join me along with his friends. My trainer, Stacey, also joined us.

Aside from having fun, the primary purpose of this race wasn't to pursue a new personal record, but to fathom how well I could handle things I am unaware of and the resultant states of ambiguity and chaos they throw me into. And given that the race was unstructured, it would present moments of confusion and the unknown that would require me to think on my feet while under pressure.

The course started uphill, and within 300 meters (984 feet) or so, we hit the first obstacle known as the spider's web, a series of crossing ropes that the participants had to navigate. Contrary to my belief that the run would be rather easy, this, the very first obstacle, troubled me quite a bit. I got caught in the yarn of the web and fell several times before making my way out of it.

The next obstacle was a muddy hole: a long water crossing with mud hills, followed by jumping into a huge square iron container filled with ice-cold water. From there, we covered a 1.5 mile of track known as Udder Chaos, with a series of obstacles to overcome. We started by climbing over a wall eight to ten feet high. Thereafter, we ran to several obstacles where we had to balance on beams, swing along monkey bars, crawl on our hands and knees through muddy pits and tunnels, and slide across a PVC pipe covered in slick lube (the Lube Tube). I conquered these obstacles with the help of Stacey, Nikhil, and other participants, especially a man who grabbed my hand and pulled me over that high wall. I know full well I could not have done this run on my own.

The mud race was an amalgam of leaping, jumping, running, jogging, slipping, sliding, crawling, balancing, climbing, and screaming with excitement. I had to use muscles that were so different from those I had used in marathons and mountain climbing. I felt exuberant, like a little boy having a great time with no parental supervision.

It was during this race that I discovered my comfort with the uncomfortable, the unknown, and the ambiguous. I had chosen curiosity and the fun of the unknown over fear. Not knowing what obstacle was coming next encouraged me to embrace the unknown, however terrifying, as ephemeral. It would pass. All I had to do was stay with it till that happened.

The Udder Mud Run was the muddiest and most unstructured

physical pursuit I had undertaken so far. All the hurdles and obstacles had to be organized to enhance the unstructured nature of the run, and the organizers had done a splendid job from start to finish.

100-Mile Bike Run, Mobile, Alabama (November 2018)

An unexciting truth may be eclipsed by a thrilling lie.

—ALDOUS HUXLEY

Marathons, mountaineering, triathlon, and the mud race had all presented great opportunities for me to try something new and push myself in ways that tested my vulnerabilities and capabilities. When confronted with the bicycle ride in the triathlon, I had to learn how to ride the speed/racing bike, and thereby found a new love for an activity I had not thought much about in the past. That had been just a thirteen mile race. Now, I was challenging myself to complete a 100-mile bike ride in a single day.

The story of my life since my bypass surgery was about ignoring the limits that medical science and age had imposed on me. Using the perseverance of the human spirit, I had exploring exhilarating and daunting activities that enabled me to experience the fullness of who I really am and discover the lessons contained within those experiences.

I had actually planned to participate in my first century bike ride in 2017, but my body deserted me. I had trained hard, starting at about five miles and gradually increasing the distance to sixty. I spread this gradual ascendancy in my endurance over about six months, until I reached the stage where I could easily bike around forty miles one day in a week.

On a very warm July day, I went out for a practice biking session and completed a forty-two-mile ride. Unfortunately, I didn't drink enough fluids during the ride. The next day, I had intense pain and pressure in my lower abdomen and I could hardly pee, emitting just a few drops of urine and blood. I knew I had acute urinary retention caused by my enlarged prostate blocking the urine flow out of my body.

I went to the emergency room. My urologist decided to fit me with a catheter in the hope that large clots of blood obstructing the urine would easily pass through. But I had to pay an unforgettable price, the torment of unbearable pain. That night was harrowing. I had to lie in one position, for if I moved even a tad, pain shot through my penis as if someone had inserted a heated iron rod into my body. The pain medications didn't help. Fortunately, the next morning, I had the catheter out and was on my way to recovery.

Everyone around me assumed it was the bike ride that had caused this. I didn't say much, even though I knew this wasn't true. However, in spite of having recovered, I had to take two months off before I started training again in October; and by November 2017, I completed 100 kilometers (62.13 miles) in a single stretch. But my heart was now set on the 100-mile bike race that would take place in Mobile, Alabama, in November 2018.

In August 2018, I started training in earnest, and by November, I had clocked close to a total of nine hundred miles. On average, I would bike three times a week on the roads of Gadsden, and sometimes on the Chief Ladiga Trail that stretches for thirty-three miles from Anniston, Alabama, to the Alabama-Georgia state line.

A week before the race, I braved the cold November weather and rode seventy miles under six hours. When I started, the temperature was 37°Fahrenheit (2.78°C), but by the time I finished, the weather had turned to a warm 62°F (16.67°C). I now felt adequately prepared for the 100-mile bike race to be held at the historic Fort Conde in downtown Mobile, Alabama.

We arrived in Mobile on Friday, the day before the race. Brutally cold weather was expected to come Mobile's way on the next day, an anomaly for us living in the South.

Saturday morning, I walked with my wife, rolling my bicycle by my side, for half a mile to Fort Conde, the starting point of the race. The going was torturously slow because of the cold wind blowing in our faces.

We had barely walked a quarter of a mile when we saw two girls biking slowly toward Fort Conde. A moment later, one of them fell off. I believe it was the wind drag and crosswinds that threw her off balance.

We went up to her to help. She had most likely sprained her ankle and decided to call it off. For a fleeting moment, I thought of giving up too. But true to my belief of accepting what cannot be controlled, I carried on.

It was biting cold at the starting point, where we had to wait for the run to start. According to some regular participants, it was the worst weather they had seen in the last ten years. To be honest, I was scared. Would I be able to handle my skinny road bike in these winds? Would I be able to bike uphill with the headwinds, or would I have to walk with my bike? What if I had to pee in this cold? Would there be enough bathroom stops?

The bike ride commenced. The extremely cold weather and winds that averaged between 10 and 20 mph meant that not only was biking uphill a tremendous challenge, going downhill was difficult because of the bone-chilling headwinds.

For cyclists, wind is the main enemy. Crosswinds have blown riders completely off the road or into the opposite traffic lane. And a small mistake in group cycling can take down a whole group of riders.

Climbing hills, each taking approximately forty minutes, was a real struggle. My speed in the headwind had dropped to a pedestrian 5–7 mph (more than half the wind speed). Combating the wind became tough. My eyes were constantly watering and burning in spite of the glasses I was wearing.

Going downhill is expected to be far easier than climbing uphill, but this time around it wasn't easy, as I had to pedal downhill in the lowest gear amid the strong winds. Contrary to many people's beliefs, coasting downhill was not an option because during windy descents, applying minimal power to the rear wheel helps the rider better control the bike.

The physical and mental demands in making such slow progress under such adverse conditions sapped some riders' motivation, and they opted to leave the race. I was tempted to follow them but managed to keep the bike upright through a line of gusty descents.

We were at the fifty-mile mark when the organizers had to reroute the next four miles. A biker had fallen on the bridge we had to cross, due to gale force winds.

The return ride was even more challenging. The ascents and descents of the windy ride in the first half of the race had taken their toll on me.

At ninety miles with only ten miles remaining, I reached the limits of my physical and mental reserves. I told Stacey that I couldn't continue.

I had slowed to a crawl and was breathing heavily. There was nothing in my body that did not hurt. My body was fatigued, and my spirits were drained. Instead of trying to motivate me with the grandeur of what I was going to achieve, Stacey lied to me. She convinced me there was a rest stop about three miles away where we could rest and decide if we wanted to carry on or abandon the race.

It was a beautiful lie. There was no rest stop after three miles, but Stacey had rekindled my motivation. I was three miles closer and had only seven miles left, which was so much better than ten. One more mile led to two, and two miles led to three. She purposefully resurrected the fire and willpower in me by having me focus on each one-mile target. I was still exhausted and in pain, but the awareness of having to complete such short distances mentally spurred me on.

It took us eight hours and forty-five minutes to complete the race. I was tired, hungry, and my butt was sore, but it didn't matter. What mattered was that, thanks to Stacey, I had completed the race and finished a century ride, a badge of honor among cyclists!

I felt ten feet tall. It was good to belong to a group of elite cyclists. But about a week after my 100-mile bike ride, I fell while trying to teach my grandson how to bike. This was in my neighborhood, near my house in Atlanta. He was about to fall off his bike, and I ran to catch him, but I fell on my face, hitting my upper front teeth on the ground. I ended up with a lip laceration, my gums bleeding, and my teeth loose and pushed inward. My dentist had to push the teeth outward to realign my bite. It was ironic that after biking nine hundred miles in four months of training and then completing the 100-mile bike ride with no injury, I hurt myself protecting my grandson just a tenth of a mile from my house.

The discomfort in my teeth lingers, but it's nothing I can't take in my stride.

Embrace the unknown. Tell a beautiful lie.

A benevolent lie that keeps someone's best interests at heart can encourage them to achieve their full potential.

6

LIVING WITH NATURE AND THRIVING WITH EXERCISE

Nature has the power to renew and refresh.

—HELEN KELLER

Eight Days in a Simple Retreat in a Small Indian Village

AS A YOUNG boy in India, I was fascinated with Edgar Rice Burroughs, the celebrated American adventure and science-fiction writer best known for creating one of the most popular characters in fiction, Tarzan. At that particular time in my life, I was fixated by this jungle hero, and often wondered how cool it would be to live in the jungle, up in a tree, with wild animals at my command.

Needless to say, that dream—like many other unrealistic dreams of youth—forever remained a dream. I don't live in a jungle, nor do I have any command over animals. When we had dogs as pets, they favored my wife's commands over mine.

But remnants of that dream must have remained in the recesses of my memories, because as I went through the ups and downs of life, I became acutely attuned to the wonders of nature and its deep connectedness with our well-being. Water to drink, food to eat, air to breathe, land to live upon are gifts of nature; and we use them to create the clothes we wear, the books we read, the comforts and the luxuries we enjoy. There isn't a single thing we can name that didn't originally come from a natural source. The first gentle rays of the sun, the trees, the fields, the meadows, and other manifestations of nature were beginning to feel as real to me as human beings.

I soon realized that I had been running marathons, climbing mountains, and jumping out of airplanes to experience the magnificence of nature around me and develop an abiding friendship with it. Or, as I like to say, "Facilitate my communion with nature." So, living outside the boundaries defined by our culture became a requirement for not only my physical well-being, but also for uplifting my mental health.

For the last ten years, I have loved being in nature for it has repeatedly exuded the power to refresh or reenergize my mind, body, and spirit. Yet like many, I have exploited nature and have been a mute spectator to increasing plunder of Earth's natural resources by us, the pampered human league.

We have gone far down the path of complete separation from nature, creating chronic anxiety and imbalance in our ambient society. As a consumer, I have seen too many of us become overly materialistic and forget the simple pleasures of life, enjoy processed garbage over growing our own food to nourish our bodies, and prefer to stay indoors in air-conditioned spaces over walking in the freshness of the morning air.

We live in a world where we patronize quick fixes. We use liposuction and laser to reduce our weight and Flex Belts to tighten our abdominal muscles, and our traditional family dinner is being increasingly replaced by take-out meals or eating-on-the-run. So, it should come as no surprise that this desire for instant gratification has permeated nearly every aspect of our lives. And I wasn't holier-than-thou. I too had developed the arrogance that generally accompanies acquiring too many material possessions and an intemperate lifestyle, until the bypass surgery sorted me out. It stirred me up a decade ago, and since then I am on the reform path.

Sometimes it takes a global crisis to enable us to go back to our roots. The coronavirus (COVID-19) pandemic is no accident. It is nature's ultimate pause and reset button. It's payback time for our destruction of this world. And as humans have retreated, nature is flourishing and reclaiming what's hers.

Since the beginning of our existence, human beings have had direct contact with nature. We are animals that started our existence in the same way as every other creature did in a natural ecosystem. It is only in the past few thousand years that we humans have developed techniques that have secluded us from our natural surroundings. Driven by external progress, we have forgotten that we are an indispensable part of nature.

In Chris Kresser's book *Unconventional Medicine*, he suggests an alternative way to deal with the root cause of chronic health conditions. He recommends reaching out to holistic practitioners from the local community who can help balance a patient's lifestyle, keeping in mind that we are an intimate part of nature and not its adversary. As postulated by the British naturalist Charles Darwin, even in our scientific experiments, we are an essential part of nature, and any experimentation has to account for the researcher's interaction in it. In other words, we do not emerge or evolve in isolation from nature in whatever course of action we take.

In a well-recognized study on this subject, environmental psychologist Roger Ulrich demonstrated that hospitalized patients recovered more quickly with a view of trees than did patients who had a view of a brick wall.

During the last few years, I have become more aware of the positive effects of nature on our wellbeing. I am now an evolving biophiliac. Across the world, communities are coming together to find a more balanced way of living. The stresses of modern life have taken their toll, and people are searching for deeper connections with each other and the natural world.

Health, mental wellness, meditation, solitude, green outdoor spaces, and the opportunity to explore natural ecosystems foster a lifelong love of nature and a curiosity about our natural habitat. In light of the growing awareness of climate change and sustainability, it is imperative for us to understand that nature is our strongest ally, and that by allowing nature to be a part of our lives, we can restore the balance in our beings.

In this context, I recount and relive my experience of living with nature for eight days at the Anahata Healing Art Center (AHAC), an Ayurveda and yoga retreat in Southern India. To those of us who live in cities, lead very busy lives, or have little opportunity to live within the splendor of nature, taking a trip every now and then to exult in the marvels of the planet can be a fulfilling time of experiencing a sense of liberating freedom and of oneness between humans and nature. You will return to your city life with a rejuvenated spirit.

From my extensive online research, AHAC seemed the right place for me to start my exploration of how nature can influence our health.

The best way to describe the intensive euphoria I experienced while at the retreat is to take you, the reader, on this journey with me. Much of what I describe was published in the May 2018 edition of the Atlanta based magazine, *Khabar*.

I started my journey from Mumbai, India. I took an early morning flight to Bengaluru (the Silicon Valley of India). From Bengaluru, it was six hours by bus to reach Mysuru, the third-largest city in the state of Karnataka. From there, I took a taxi to Ravundur, a small, sleepy village about two hours from Mysuru. A total of 655 families reside in Ravundur. There was plenty to reflect upon as my old, rickety taxi bounced along the dirt road through pastoral farmlands.

There was a characteristic beauty and simple charm to the farms and villages I passed—farmers plowing their fields, feeding their cattle and milking their cows, women pounding rice and carrying water on their heads, and scantily-clad children playing. They all seemed happy and contented.

Upon our arrival in the village, my driver had a hard time finding the center, but the friendly locals guided us by pointing toward a narrow street that led to the entrance of AHAC. Kiran, the owner of the retreat, met me at the entrance, which had a table and two benches set on one side. Nothing identified the center to a passerby. For a moment, I froze. Had I really come to the right place?

Kiran took the time to explain what AHAC provided for its guests. Being part of the community, the retreat played an important role in giving back, particularly to kids with special needs and marginalized groups. After our initial chat, he led me to my room. I removed my shoes outside before entering the sparsely furnished room. In spite of Kiran's warning, "Come with no expectations," I was shocked when I first saw the meager state of the room. First, an uninviting entrance, and now this ordinary room. I had stayed in places far worse than this, up in the mountains and on the Kailash yatra, but this was astonishingly pared down to the minimum. Yet, for some inexplicable reason, I didn't walk out.

Kiran bid good-bye to me for the night with this simple, laid-back philosophy, which I paraphrase: "There is no rush. Sleep well and observe what is going around the grounds of the retreat in the morning. You can then decide if this is something you would be interested in and would like to support. There is no request or compulsion to support anything."

That nonchalant statement created the most liberating feeling I had experienced in years. This sense of uninhibited freedom and flow set the tone of my incredible experiences at the center.

Life at AHAC was different each day, and we were encouraged to be spontaneous. There were no tasks lists or timetables to adhere to. You just wake up and take it one day at a time. The initial lack of structure and goals were a shock to me, coming from the United States where we make planning a priority. But I realized that once you let go of your expectations, you are more likely to accept things that just happen. I opted to try colon cleansing for the first few days (clear juices the first day, followed by fruits the next day, and purging the third day).

Typically, our day started with yoga at the retreat or at the local temple, which was a short walk from AHAC. The ringing of the temple bells was our wake-up call as the sun rose majestically, coaxing us to get into the yoga flow. Birds sang, perched in the abundance of trees surrounding us. The red clayish soil soaked with morning dew gave forth an earthy smell that, to me, was far better than any fragrance sold in the Western world.

The entire experience was mesmerizing. Back to the roots, to the soulful, calm, and harmonious rhythm of nature, part of an authentic Indian village miles away from the automated, busy, restless, and modern mode of life. A great place to slow down, reflect, and reconnect with nature. The air of peace, simplicity, and tranquility enabled me to reset my body and mind.

After yoga, we would stroll through the streets of the village, where we interacted with men from the local community. We joined them for chats over coffee that was served in tiny cups. These conversations were lively, friendly, interesting, and varied. Topics ranged from business, health, politics, our hometowns, and the most popular sport in India, cricket, a bat-and-ball game that evokes intense passion and strong opinions, similar to the fervor experienced among people watching the Super Bowl in the United States.

After our animated discussions, we would return to AHAC to help in the kitchen or in weeding the garden, or just relax in the communal area. We were then served breakfast, which was traditionally cooked, yet healthy and tasty. I found that eating natural foods provided clarity of thinking and a sense of inner calm.

Jean Anthelme Brillat-Savarin, the French gastronome, observed, "Tell me what you eat and I will tell you what you are." The center provided us whole-food, plant-based vegetarian meals that consisted of organic fruits, vegetables, grains, and herbs that were sourced onsite at their farm. Lunch consisted of Indian flat bread (made from rice and whole-wheat flour), chickpeas, parsley, onion, tomato, and cumin with coconut or coriander sauce (chutney). Pongal, a popular South Indian dish, was served at dinner. It is made of rice, yellow lentils, curry leaves, cashews, turmeric, black pepper, cumin seeds, and ginger paste.

In the afternoon, we mingled with local workers, helping them to plant trees or carry water from a nearby water pool; or we read or meditated in the natural surroundings. There was a school nearby bustling with the sounds of children playing and school bells ringing. These were soothing sounds.

I was fascinated to watch men and women work together in harmony to build an outdoor sun area for the elderly, without the use of modern tools, while still making time to smile and chat in the hot midday sun. The materials they used were natural—palm leaves and wood—except for the plastic tarpaulins to make it waterproof. There was also a functioning swimming pool made of rocks and stones.

Ongoing projects included the construction of new rooms made with natural materials, such as mud, water, and wood. For AHAC, it was important to be as self-sustaining as possible without adversely affecting the environment around the center. These rooms were for older people in the community who could not look after themselves. Volunteers from the community took turns bringing them food and helping them around. I met a lady who had been bedridden for two years until she was brought there. She is now able to walk for a few minutes a day without any modern surgical intervention.

As I reflect upon it, the retreat imparted the warm and inviting feeling of a community that contributes to the needs of others and instills a sense of camaraderie, trust, belonging, and partnership for a common purpose. It certainly was a way of life there—to be cared for and to reciprocate that caring.

My peers at the center were from different countries. Maureen and Will from the United Kingdom, Lance from Canada, Keiko from Japan, and Laura from Germany, all volunteers there. Will and I did a few 5K runs around the fields. What a remarkably different experience it was. One evening, we decided to walk to a nearby village, and a farmer on his tractor stopped and gave us a ride. It was customary for the locals to stop their scooters and ask if any walking tourists needed a ride.

We visited several houses in the vicinity, and the people not only opened their homes to us, but also their hearts. Despite the spartan living conditions and few possessions, their faces lit up with genuine and welcoming smiles. They cooked simple but delicious meals for us. The offering was made unreservedly, with no expectation of wanting anything in return. I could only reciprocate by sharing my medical knowledge with them and answering questions that came my way. The simple village folk taught me that even with less, they give more. Their generous hearts are willing to share. Therein lies their secret to happiness.

Just before bedtime, we got together in the communal area and talked about our experiences of the day and what we could take back home. We hit the sack, already accustomed to dogs barking, letting sleep overtake our tired but fulfilled minds and bodies.

Nature is our strongest ally

For a healthy, happy, and meaningful life, you can take small steps to make nature an indispensable part of your life. Try jogging or walking in a natural environment as opposed to walking or running on a treadmill at home or in the gymnasium. Spending more time outside in green, natural spaces will leave you more attentive, energized, and happier than exercising indoors.

If you live in a city, it may take some effort to find a quiet tree-lined path to walk, jog, or ride a bike, or perhaps to read a book in peace. But try to discover a park, trail, or playground. If you have proprietorship of any land—for instance, on the terrace—you could do some gardening. This can be made into a routine by setting regular times to tend to your plants. It's a great way to reduce stress levels, lift your mood, and relax the mind.

When walking, running, or playing an outdoor sport, you will become conscious of being one with nature (in whatever small way), and this feeling is a wonderful complement to the physical well-being that you will derive from the exercise. Connecting with nature and befriending it will also improve your mental health.

Nature provides us all the resources we need to survive and progress. Enjoy it, feel it, draw energy from it, care for it, and respect it, and it will give you the gift of an unusually healthy and happy life.

7

DIET IS MORE IMPORTANT
THAN EXERCISE

*No disease that can be treated with diet should be treated with
any other means.*

—MOSES MAIMONIDES

Egg, Meat, Dairy, and Sugar: Four Biggest Adversaries of Your Health

Had I known then what I know and believe today, I would not have undergone the stents (age fifty-six) or the bypass surgery (age sixty-one). I would have cured or healed my heart disease by following a whole-food, plant-based (WFPB) diet.

This is not to say that a coronary angioplasty (including stenting) or a bypass surgery is not to be performed at all. It is, but only in an emergency medical condition.

As a doctor, recovered bypass surgery patient, mountaineer, marathoner, consumer of food products, and as someone who has tried various diets—compulsive carnivore, flexitarian (primarily vegetarian or plant-based foods with the occasional indulgence of meat or fish), pescatarian (a vegetarian diet that includes fish and seafood), junk food vegetarian (replacing meat, dairy, and eggs with refined and processed foods), and finally a whole-food, plant-based diet—I can say with conviction that a WFPB diet can reverse heart diseases, improve cholesterol, and lower blood pressure.

I have had my fair share of ailments in my life, and these are mostly of my own making: high cholesterol, enlarged prostate resulting in acute urinary retention, chronic constipation, heart disease, and a perforated colon due to severe diverticulitis, to name a few. It is a standing joke in my clinic that when a patient lists his or her medical problems, I can remark, "Don't worry, I have had these problems too."

The idea of a WFPB diet that I highly recommend may not be easy to accept, particularly for meat eaters and vegetarians who consider it their staple diet. *An unhealthy vegetarian diet is just as bad as consuming the flesh of any animal (red meat, poultry, and seafood).* Just because a product is labeled vegetarian doesn't mean it's healthier than a meat-based food.

This detailed chapter is my earnest attempt to convince some, if not many, readers to try to follow a plant-based diet. I won't merely state how such a diet is good for you, but will relate it to my experiences and perspectives as a physician, former heart-disease patient, and consumer. I will also support my argument with suitable research, references, and relevant information.

Besides the data and evidence offered in this chapter, which I have attempted to present in a reader-friendly manner, I also touch on some significant nonscientific aspects of a healthy diet. These include fad diets, the connection between financial well-being and physical health, and why a high percentage of doctors, despite knowing what is *right from wrong,* still treat the consequence of a disease and not the disease itself.

Death is a universal certainty. Good health eases and facilitates the pathway to death by allowing us to enjoy our life fully and make the most of our time on planet Earth. This is possible only when we increase our ability to be fully functional and avoid disabling, painful, and lengthy battles with disease. This fact is corroborated by the book *The China Study Revised and Expanded Edition: The Most Comprehensive Study of Nutrition Ever Conducted and the Startling Implications for Diet, Weight*

Loss, and Long-Term Health by T. Colin Campbell, PhD, and Thomas M. Campbell II, MD), which states on page 75, "There are many better ways to die and to live."

Fifteen years ago, when I first confronted health problems, I decided to overcome them by practicing yoga and other forms of regular exercise. But there was something missing. How could I solve my eternal problems with bowel movements and also avoid further heart problems?

I mention bowel movements because I have found older patients who are admitted for major surgery are often more worried about their bowel movements than the surgery itself. Further, in spite of my daily exercise, I still felt I needed to do more for my heart to make it stronger. To understand more about the functioning of our bodies in terms of nutrition, I turned to the extensive research and study on the subject done by nutrition experts, namely Neal Barnard, MD, Nandita Shah, Caldwell B. Esselstyn Jr., MD, Dean Ornish, MD, T. Colin Campbell, PhD, Thomas M. Campbell II, MD, and Michael Greger, MD.

I decided to deal with my heart disease first, as this is the biggest killer in the United States, India, and many other countries. As I understood diet and nutrition better, I gave up meat but occasionally ate fish. The next thing I quit was dairy. Being lactose intolerant, I really didn't care for it. Then I stopped eating eggs, and finally I cut fish from my diet. But at the back of my mind, I was nervous.

As an athlete, I was worried plant-based protein wouldn't be enough. I was also concerned about my performance time (time taken to prepare for a race) and my recovery time after a race, including healing after an injury.

At first, consuming a large piece of chicken or fish after each long run was a must, and it became a habit that I thoroughly enjoyed. But after each race, it would take me at least five to seven days to recover. Why? Was I overdoing it, or was it something else?

I distinctly remember the 100-kilometer (62.13 miles) bike ride that I completed in November 2017 with my friend and trainer, Stacey. I was a vegan then, abstaining from meat, eggs, dairy products, and other animal-derived ingredients. After finishing the bike ride, we stopped at a restaurant, and I had a vegetarian meal. Our plan was to stay overnight and travel the next morning. But I felt so good that we decided to drive back to Gadsden that night, a four-hour drive. Halfway into the drive, I got a call from my clinic that the doctor who was supposed to work the next day had called in sick. The following morning, I took his place and worked ten hours straight like it was any other day.

It was then that I wondered what I was doing differently that made me feel so energetic. The only thing different was that I was now eating a whole-food, plant-based diet. I have, since then, run several 5Ks and 10Ks, as well as finished a 100-mile bike race (November 2018). After careful deliberation, I realized—although this is not scientifically based—that that was the only significant change I had made. I attributed the extra energy to my plant-based diet. I now knew and understood that *diet is more important than exercise*, and I am a living proof to that.

Here are the reasons for dietary concern: artery blockages, angina pain, sudden heart attack, and death. For most of us on a conventional American diet, we form fatty deposits in the walls of the coronary arteries just like we make consistent deposits to a savings account to accumulate money. These deposits develop over decades, gradually narrowing the walls of the arteries and the path of the blood flow to the heart. This restriction of blood flow leads to chest pain during exercise or exertion, referred to by doctors as angina.

Recent scientific evidence, however, indicates that most heart attacks occur when younger, soft, friable fatty plaques (fatty deposits) rupture and bleed, forming a blood clot in the artery which causes sudden blockage of the blood supply to a certain part of the heart. This is catastrophic, and 50 percent of people who have a heart attack die within an hour. This is referred to as sudden, unexpected cardiac death or cardiac arrest by doctors. *Both my clinic partners, who are doctors, have had heart attacks with less than 50 percent blockages.*

On the other hand, in angina, the plaques are generally large and contain scar tissue and calcium, which makes them sturdier, unlikely to break and cause a heart attack.[3] I had angina and not a heart attack. Two of my coronary arteries were more than 90 percent blocked. I never encountered sudden, sharp chest pain, shortness of breath, or sweating, which would have suggested a heart attack.

"A large, international study led by Stanford and New York University found that invasive procedures are no better than medications and lifestyle advice at treating heart disease that's severe but stable.[4]

John P. Cooke, MD, PhD, Professor of Medicine (Cardiovascular Medicine), Emeritus at Stanford University, acknowledges that angioplasty, while it helps relieve angina, hardly ever saves lives, and does nothing whatsoever to cure heart disease. *"He suggests, in fact, that about half of all angioplasties done in the US each year are simply unnecessary. The same goes for bypass surgeries. It is far better to restore the health of your endothelium, i.e., the inner lining of the coronaries that produces nitric oxide that helps dilate the blood vessels and protects the wall of the arteries. In this context, it is almost always better to try a medical approach in conjunction with a dietary approach to restore the health of the endothelium."*[5]

In the West, particularly in the United States, gluttony became an unstoppable phenomenon primarily because of the easy availability of food, which led to an epidemic of obesity. *"The age-adjusted prevalence of obesity among US adults was 42.4 percent in 2017-2018. There was no significant difference in the prevalence of obesity between men and women overall or by age group."*[6]

Over the years, all kinds of weight-loss diets have popped up like mushrooms, some focusing on reducing one's appetite, others restricting calories, carbohydrates (carbs), and/or fats. But it is apparent that this manifestation of our bodies based on what we eat has side effects on young people—mostly girls but also boys—who end up binge eating, followed by self-induced vomiting, purging, or fasting. While the market continues to promote scores of diets, some of them rely not so much on good health factor but on foods that make the body look good.

And while the debate rages on about what is the best diet for human beings, it is becoming increasingly clear that exercising the body and mind together with a diet that leans toward the whole-food, plant-based is the key to vitality and longevity. Furthermore, it's conducive to maintaining a body structure that would be the envy of our predecessors and will improve the quality of our lives. We are, however, far from achieving this.

While people in both developed and developing countries are living longer than generations before them, the extra years are not healthy ones. *We are living longer but sicker; we are living longer but not necessarily healthier.* In the United States, there is a large dependency on drugs in attempts to alleviate the pain and suffering of a bedridden patient.

"Nearly 70 percent of Americans are on at least one prescription drug, and more than half take two, Mayo Clinic and Olmsted Medical Center researchers say."[7] Being dependent on prescription drugs for chronic conditions like heart disease, diabetes, high blood pressure, and cholesterol can be avoided if we start eating right. According to Dr. Michael Greger, MD, author of *How Not to Die*, "According to the most rigorous analysis of risk factors ever published,[1] the number one cause of death and disability in the United States is our diet."[8]

People of South Asian Descent and Heart Disease

Heart disease is the leading cause of death in India, the United States, as well as in the world overall. People of South Asian descent, which includes countries like India, Pakistan, Nepal, Sri Lanka, Bangladesh, Bhutan, and Maldives, will most likely tell you they have close relatives who have heart disease or have died unexpectedly of a heart attack.

"South Asians represent about a quarter of the world's population, yet it account for about 60 percent of heart disease patients."[9]

According to the Stanford South Asian Translational Heart Initiative (SSATHI), "In the United States, South Asians have a four times greater risk of heart disease than the general population and have a much greater chance of having a heart attack before age 50. 25 percent of heart attacks occur under age 40 for young South Asians, and 50 percent occur under age 50."

This may seem like a huge contradiction, because it is common knowledge that people from these countries do not consume as much meat and meat products as do people elsewhere in the world.

A cohort of US South Asians called Mediators of Atherosclerosis in

---

1 According to the Global Burden of Disease study, the largest study of human risk factors for disease in history, funded by the Bill and Melinda Gates Foundation, "The number one cause of death in the United States is our diet."

South Asians Living in America (MASALA) found that 40 percent of its participants are vegetarian. Vegetarianism is a common practice in India, and it is widely regarded in the West as heart healthy. But vegetarians who consume traditional South Asian foods like fried snacks, sweetened beverages, and high-fat dairy products were found to have worse cardiovascular health than those who eat what the researchers call a "prudent" diet, with more fruits, vegetables, nuts, beans, and whole grains.[10]

South Asians have a cultural and emotional connection to oil and clarified butter (ghee). When we serve food or entertain our family and friends, adding more oil or ghee to the food is considered a sign of warmth and generosity. So, when the pot of curry or the pan of vegetables does not have oil floating on the top, it indicates the food is not tasty because you are being stingy with the oil or clarified butter.

We have a predisposition to Type 2 diabetes and high blood pressure, and tend to carry higher levels of triglycerides (a type of fat found in the blood) and lower levels of good cholesterol. I have observed this among my South Asian patients, and it is confirmed by the American Heart Association: "Ethnicity a 'risk-enhancing' factor under new cholesterol guidelines" by American Heart Association News, January 11, 2019.

Also, recent findings of high levels of coronary artery calcium—a marker of atherosclerosis, which is the narrowing or blocking of the arteries—was found in South Asians, and this can be an early harbinger of future heart attacks and strokes.[11]

South Asians are not normally associated with being overweight or obese, and they do not use much tobacco, common risk factors for heart diseases. Our body mass index (BMI) is generally normal. (BMI is calculated by taking a person's weight and dividing it by the square of his or her height.) A healthy BMI range is between 18.5 and 24.9. A BMI of 25 to 29.9 is classified as overweight, and someone with a BMI of 30 or over is considered obese. But South Asians do carry fat. According to a MASALA study of 1,164 South Asian women and men aged 40-84 years, *South Asians have a lot of visceral fat in the abdominal area, the liver, and around the heart.* It is this visceral fat that is directly related to heart disease. So, it is better to consider BMI levels of 22.9 and below as normal, 23 to 27 as overweight, and over 27 as obese. Also, it is best to calculate your waist circumference to get a better idea of visceral fat. The normal waist circumference is 35 inches in males and 30 inches in females.

In the same study by MASALA, it was found that the fat around the heart and in the body cavity had the strongest association with heart disease risk, followed by the fat in the muscle. Fat under the skin is considered the primary location of fat in healthy normal-weight individuals that is generally not seen in South Asians.

As I have said before, eating a healthy diet and exercising can offset genetic predisposition. But South Asians are not physically active (barring exceptions, we don't do any serious exercise), and this is quite noticeable, especially as it relates to first-generation South Asians in America. Regular exercise also increases your good cholesterol and protects your heart.

Finally, South Asians may be aware of the risk of heart disease but seldom talk about it. What an irony! You can talk about your son or daughter getting into medical school, but you cannot talk about how your son just had a heart attack.

It is never too late to start a heart-healthy diet. Dr. Dean Ornish (www.ornish.com), an American physician and researcher, took patients with advanced heart disease and put them on a WFPB diet with no oil or fat from any external source. His hope was to stop or halt the progression of heart disease. But better still, his patient's heart disease started to reverse (restoration of endothelium by diet). Dean Ornish is the president and founder of the nonprofit Preventive Medicine Research Institute in Sausalito, California, and a clinical professor of medicine at the University of California, San Francisco.

According to Ajai R. Singh and Shakuntala A. Singh, editors of Mens Sana Monographs, "Sicknesses are not reducing in number. They are changing in type. If infectious diseases and malnutrition took their toll in the earlier centuries (and in certain sections of the world even today), lifestyle diseases, chronic conditions, and neoplastic disorders are taking their toll in the present. It is almost like changing fashions in the world of disease."[12]

What Can You Do to Prevent Heart Disease Risk?

- Become aware of your family health history and act on it.
- Talk to a doctor who knows about the heart disease risks South Asians carry.
- Exercise thirty minutes (under stress-free conditions) six days a week.
- Eat heart-healthy food. Add more fruits, vegetables, legumes, nuts, beans, and whole grains to your diet. Reduce simple carbohydrates (simple sugars like glucose, fructose, and sucrose) and increase your complex carbohydrates (whole grains and starchy vegetables).
- Bring yoga, spirituality, and meditation into your life.

Remember, eating an unhealthy vegetarian diet is just as bad as consuming the flesh of any animal (red meat, poultry, and seafood).

Disease and Genetics

Back in 1903, Thomas Edison predicted, "The doctor of the future will give no medicine, but will instruct his patient in the care of (the) human frame in diet and in the cause and prevention of diseases."

But this is the twenty-first century. Many people strongly believe diseases and death are programmed in our genes. However, for most of the leading causes of death, science shows that our genes account for only 10–20 percent of risk, at most. Even if you do have a high genetic risk, a healthy plant-based diet is capable of negating most, if not all, of the risk by controlling the gene expression (gene regulation). It is not bad genes that run in the family, it is bad diet that runs in the family.

Then there are people who believe that if you have good genes, you can eat indiscriminately, skip exercise, and nothing will happen to you. I, for one, believed so. My paternal grandfather died at the ripe old age of 102, and my father died at the age of eighty-three. I was foolish to believe the good-genes theory. I had my first angioplasty with stents at the age of fifty-six and my open-heart bypass surgery at sixty-one.

The rates of chronic diseases, including cancer, differ significantly among various populations around the globe. However, when people move from low-risk to high-risk countries, their disease rates almost always change to those of the new environment. New country, new culture, new environment, and a new lifestyle will most likely change your diet. And a new diet means new diseases. Studies have shown that Japanese who moved to America and started the American diet had the same rate of heart disease as their American counterparts.

Eating Habits and Incidence of Chronic Diseases

During the 1930s and1940s, hospitals in sub-Saharan Africa noticed there were no chronic Western diseases such as high blood pressure, diabetes, heart disease, and strokes in the local population. It was not because these people were dying early of other diseases, or never living long enough to develop heart disease. When comparisons were made through autopsies between Ugandans and Americans dying at the same age, it was found that among 632 Americans autopsied, 136 had heart attacks, while in the 632 Ugandans autopsied, there was only a single heart attack.[13] The book *The China Study* attributed this to the rural population in sub-Saharan Africa having very low cholesterol levels.

In fact, studies show that if the total cholesterol is under 150 and the low-density lipoprotein (LDL) cholesterol (bad cholesterol) is under 70, there is a high risk of developing coronary artery disease (CAD), also called coronary heart disease (CHD).

Prominent heart disease researchers and physicians, Drs. William Castelli, William Roberts, and Caldwell Esselstyn Jr., "in their long careers have never seen a heart disease fatality among their patients who had blood cholesterol levels below 150mg/dL."[14]

So why were the cholesterol levels in the rural population of sub-Saharan Africa so low? It was most likely their diet. They lived on a WFPB diet of leafy greens, root vegetables, and beans. Maize, millet rice, couscous, yams, and bananas were eaten as main meals; or alternatively, they ate porridges (oats or oatmeal) and sides. In comparison, the American diet in the studied sample consisted of meat, fish, eggs, and dairy.

In essence, three basic methods of significantly reducing bad cholesterol (LDL) are:

1. Avoid foods with trans fats (processed foods, meat, and dairy).

2. Avoid foods with saturated fats (animal foods and junk foods).

3. Avoid foods sensitive to dietary cholesterol (meats, fish, eggs, and dairy).

As people attain financial stability or build wealth, they change their eating habits and lifestyles. Wealth enables them to buy food products they could not afford in the past.

Since animal products, generally speaking, are more expensive, they become the desired food for people who now have the means to buy them. In other words, they follow in the steps of the affluent, regardless of how healthy their previous diet may have been. Thus, as wealth increases, more people on average die from diseases attributed to consuming animal products than those who cannot afford to purchase them.

Heart-related problems are often considered as *diseases of affluence* because they are tightly linked to eating habits. However, eating *right* not only helps promote a healthy heart. It also protects you from a host of other ailments that have direct linkage with dietary factors, including impotence; arthritis; obesity; diabetes; cancers of the breasts, prostate, and colon; and possibly cognitive impairment (dementia) that may strike later in life. And if you eat for good health, a major side benefit is, "You will never have to count calories or worry about your weight for the rest of your life."[15]

As I stated earlier, mainstream medicine treats the consequences of a disease, and can thereby offer instant or tremendous relief, but it does nothing to treat the underlying cause of the disease. It is like mopping the floor around an overflowing sink instead of simply turning off the faucet.

Curative cure or curative health (to cure people after they get sick) takes up 57 percent of the money spent on health care, while a mere 3 percent is spent on preventative measures.[16]

If treating the cause is safer, cheaper, and better, then why don't we doctors do so?

Because we doctors aren't trained for it. Medical schools do not spend adequate time enlightening students with courses on the effects of proper nutrition, exercise, and meditation. The National Academy of Sciences recommends only twenty-five hours of nutritional courses out of the 2,047 hours needed to receive a medical degree. Sixty percent of medical schools offer even less than twenty-five hours.[17]

Food plays such an important role in our lives, and yet most doctors give scant attention to it. Is it because doctors don't get reimbursed for such health recommendations? Money is a powerful determinant in medical practice and research. Suffice to say, if I had to start my medical practice all over again, I would be a pauper because my focus would be on treating the cause of the disease and not as much the consequences of the disease.

It is my contention that had I been taught to treat the causes of chronic illnesses like heart disease, diabetes, high blood pressure, and high cholesterol, it would not only have benefited the patient, but I could have saved a lot of money for the health-care system as well.

As alluded earlier, a diet that best prevents and treats the above conditions is a WFPB diet; i.e., the consumption of unrefined plant foods, which discourages meat, dairy, eggs, and processed refined foods.

Eating a meaty, fat-saturated diet is so ingrained in the American system that I have often heard people say there is no reason for them to change if they are leading a healthy life. These people base their decision on a gamble that diseases such as high blood pressure or diabetes will never affect their lives negatively. This cavalier attitude is exacerbated by the fact that they agree to take medicines and turn vegetarian when they are unexpectedly impacted by such diseases.

In many Americans, however, atherosclerosis starts at age eight when a person eats a typical American diet, and you may not even be lucky enough to survive your first heart attack, based on the fact that *"Sudden cardiac death (SCD) is often the first expression of coronary art disease (CAD) and is responsible for approximately 50 percent of deaths from CAD."*[18] Besides, you may not be aware you have high blood pressure or diabetes until you develop medical complications from these diseases. And then, as already mentioned, you will be put on medication that will keep you alive but will not help you lead a healthy life.

The obvious conclusion from my discussions above is to reiterate that the emphasis needs to be not to cure a disease but to prevent a disease.

In medical schools, students learn there are three levels of preventive medicine. The first is primary prevention, as in preventing people at risk of heart disease from suffering a first heart attack. So, your doctor may give you cholesterol-lowering drugs, if you have high cholesterol. The second level of prevention is when you already have a disease, say a heart attack, and you are trying to prevent a second heart attack. Your doctor may now prescribe aspirin and other medications. The third level of prevention focuses on helping people manage long-term health problems, so your doctor may prescribe a cardiac rehabilitation program to prevent further physical deterioration and pain.

The doctor may also put you on an antidepressant if you are depressed. (In my medical practice, most of the patients become depressed after a heart attack or a major surgery. I was no exception. After I had stents inserted, I was afflicted with severe depression and required psychotherapy and antidepressants.)

In the year 2000, a fourth level was proposed that would reduce the complications from the drugs and surgery of the first three levels. It had first been introduced by the World Health organization in 1978. Decades later, it was finally embraced by the American Heart Association (AHA).

But there is a fifth level of prevention, appropriately called the primordial prevention, which not very many people want to talk about. This levels addresses not just preventing chronic disease but preventing the risk factors that lead to chronic disease. For example, instead of preventing someone with high cholesterol from having a heart attack, why not prevent the person from developing high cholesterol in the first place?

With this in mind, the AHA came up with Life's Simple 7, the factors that can lead to a healthier life: stop smoking, maintain a healthy weight (lose weight by burning more calories than you eat), manage blood pressure (stress and poor diet are linked to high blood pressure), reduce blood sugar (limit sweets and sugary beverages), control cholesterol (eat smart and exercise adequately), get active (defined as walking thirty minutes a day), and eat healthier (a diet full of fruits and vegetables).

Their aim was to reduce heart disease by 20 percent by the year 2020. If 90 percent of the heart attacks can be prevented by lifestyle changes, why aim for only 20 percent? This is because most people have a hard time following a diet.

"An analysis of the health behaviors of thirty-five thousand adults across the United States was published in the Journal of the American Heart Association."[19] Most of them got a passing score in all of the above factors except diet. The diets were scored on a scale of one to five. Only 1 percent of the participants reached a healthy eating score of four. This lends veracity to my argument that if you eat a WFPB diet and are physically active, you are in safe hands, as those two factors can take care of almost all the above seven factors.

Egg, Meat, Dairy, and Sugar: Four Biggest Adversaries of Your Health

A. Egg and Meat: Plant-based protein versus animal-based protein

Upon further introspection in correlating my health problems with the food I ate, I realized that egg, meat, dairy, and sugar are the biggest adversaries to one's good health, particularly as it pertains to animal proteins.

Animal and plant proteins contain the essential amino acids our bodies require, but plant protein contains a lower portion of these amino acids. Consuming a higher proportion of amino acids may damage your health. How much protein should one eat per day? "As per Healthline, you should take 0.36 grams of protein per pound of body weight."[20]

The amount of protein in a single eight-ounce steak is about seventy grams, which far exceeds the Institute of Medicine's (IOM) daily requirement of fifty-six grams for an average sedentary man and forty-six grams for an average sedentary woman. Protein deficiency is almost unheard of in the United States. With the traditional Western diet, the average American consumes about double the protein their body needs.

Thus, the quality of plant protein is not in question (as some people have suggested). What is important is the proportional intake of amino acid (based on body weight and other considerations), which is very high in animal products and much lower in plant-based diets. It's easy to get all the protein you need without eating meat, dairy, and eggs. A variety of legumes (beans, peas, and lentils) and vegetables can provide all the essential amino acids your body needs.

Following are findings from some of my research on several ways animal proteins can damage your health:

1. Animal protein lacks fiber

   Plant protein comes packed with fiber, while animal proteins, such as eggs, meat, fish, poultry, and dairy, have no fiber. Fiber intake is associated with decreased cancer risk (colon and breast), lower risk of ulcerative colitis, diverticulitis, constipation, and Crohn's disease. "The Institute of Medicine recommends that adults eat 38 grams of fiber, but on an average, adults in the United States only eat 15 grams."[21]

2. Animal protein and cancer linkage

   "Certain proteins in meat, fish, and poultry cooked at high temperatures, especially grilling and frying, produce heterocyclic amines (chemicals formed when meat is cooked at high temperatures). These substances have been linked to various cancers, including those of the colon and breast."[22]

3. Animal protein and reduced kidney function

   When people eat too much animal protein, nitrogen is released in the blood, or it is digested and metabolized. This puts a strain on the kidneys, as they have to expel the waste through urine. High-protein diets are associated with reduced kidney functions, and over time, may lead to permanent loss of kidney function. Harvard Medical School researchers reported recently that high-protein diets were associated with a significant decline in kidney function, based on observations in 1,624 women participating in the Nurses' Health Study.

The good news is that the damage was found only in those who already had reduced kidney function at the study's outset. The bad news is that as many as one in four adults in the United States may already have reduced kidney function, suggesting that most people who have renal problems are unaware of that fact and do not realize that high-protein diets may put them at risk for further deterioration.

The American Academy of Family Physicians notes that the high intake of animal proteins can be responsible in part "for the high prevalence of kidney stones in the United States and other developed countries, and recommends protein restriction for prevention of recurrent kidney stones."[23]

4. Animal protein and Trimethylamine N-oxide (TMAO)
   Consuming animal protein that is considered high in choline can cause certain bacteria in the gut to turn choline into trimethylamine (TMA), which is absorbed in our systems and oxidized to turn into TMAO.

   TMAO is the substance that injures the lining of our blood vessels, creates inflammation, and enhances the formation of cholesterol plaques in our blood vessels.[24]

   According to the past president of American College of Cardiology, Dr. Kim A. Williams, "this one issue (TMAO), even without all the other risks associated with eating animal foods, is, in his opinion, sufficient to recommend 100 percent plant-based vegan diets."[25]

5. Animal protein increase cholesterol
   Most animal proteins contain saturated fat and cholesterol. Humans do not need to consume any cholesterol since our body synthesizes all the cholesterol we need for physiological functions. Cholesterol and saturated fats increase the risk of "heart disease, which is the leading cause of death for men, women, and people of most racial and ethnic groups in the United States."[26]

6. Animal protein can lead to osteoporosis
    High animal protein intake is known to increase urinary loss of calcium, which can lead to osteoporosis, a condition in which bones become weak and brittle. Plant-based diets with adequate proteins can significantly lower the risk of osteoporosis. We can get adequate calcium from plant foods, including leafy green vegetables, from beans and some nuts and seeds, as well as from fortified fruit juices, cereals, and non-dairy milk.[27]

7. Heme iron induces production of carcinogens
    Iron is the most abundant metal in the human body. We can consume it in two forms: *heme iron*, found primarily in animal foods like meat, poultry, and fish; and *non-heme iron*, found widely in plant foods. High intake of heme iron has been associated with many kinds of gastrointestinal cancers as well as other pathologies.[28]

    High protein diets for weight loss, disease prevention, and enhanced athletic performance have been greatly publicized in recent years. Since foods are a package deal, Dr. Walter Willett, the Fredrick John Stare Professor of Epidemiology and Nutrition at the Harvard School of Public Health opines, "We emphasize plant sources of protein, rather than animal sources."[29] Most of the other nutrients packaged with plant proteins may positively influence our long-term health as opposed to animal protein.

B. Dairy

In the animal kingdom, no species other than humans drink milk once they are weaned. We are also the only species that drinks milk of another species. Joaquin Phoenix, Academy Award winner for best actor in a leading role for *Joker*, said in his 2020 Oscar acceptance speech, "We feel entitled to artificially inseminate a cow, and when she gives birth, we steal her baby, even though her cries of anguish are unmistakable. Then we take her milk that's intended for her calf, and we put it in our coffee and our cereal."

The mamas are often heard mooing helplessly into the night in the hope of hearing from their babies. The calves are taken away, locked in tiny crates, force-fed, slaughtered, and sold as veal. But the vintage '80s commercial—*"Milk ... It Does A Body Good"*— promoted the idea that drinking milk leads to healthy bones and increased strength. Even now, some pediatricians confirm that milk is needed in children's diets, as it provides essential nutrients for them to grow up healthy.

Here are several reasons why we should avoid dairy. Andrew Olson, creator of One Ingredient Chef, published an important blog post titled, "10 Reasons to Get Your Milk From Nuts Instead of Cows." *Six of the ten reasons* are appended below. It validates my argument that dairy products should be eschewed.

1. Hormones
   As with most other mammals, cows only lactate when pregnant, and are thus kept pregnant nearly constantly. This leads to incredible levels of estrogen.

   On top of that, they are also injected with even more hormones to produce much more milk than they ever could naturally. Estrogen is closely tied to cancers of the breasts, ovaries, and prostates.[30]

   "It is no surprise then that men who consume more dairy products are 30 percent more likely to develop prostate cancer than men who consume little or no dairy."[31]

2. Saturated fat
   Dairy is the single largest source of saturated fat in our diet. At least one-third of all saturated fat consumed in America comes from cheese, butter, milk, and other dairy-based products. Given that saturated fat is a primary cause of heart disease and obesity, it doesn't seem so smart to chug glass after glass of this "liquid meat," as Rip Esselstyn (an American health activist and food writer) likes to call it in his book *The Engine 2 Seven-Day Rescue Diet: Eat Plants, Lose Weight, Save Your Health.* He further states that an ounce of beef has about the same amount of fatty acids and cholesterol as a cup of 2 percent milk.

3. Humans are lactose intolerant

"Humans were not designed to suck on the udders of bovine creatures. We're not even designed to ingest the milk of our own species after the first few years of life."[32] "This is likely why the majority of humans (over 60 percent) are incapable of fully digesting lactose,"[33] the main sugar found in milk.

Dairy products contain casein, a protein that calves can digest but that creates problems in humans. If you ever thought of giving up dairy, it probably crossed your mind at least once that you might not be able to live without cheese. Cheese addiction is real, and once you break from it, the cravings stop.

As casein breaks down, it releases casomorphins, opioids that belong to the same family of drugs, such as morphine and opium, that induce euphoric feelings and lower pain. But just as with morphine and opium, casomorphins are addictive. If you suddenly stop eating cheese (which has a very high concentration of casomorphins: it takes ten pounds of milk to make one pound of cheese), you might suffer from uncomfortable withdrawal symptoms and strong cravings.

Besides, as Dr. Frank Lipman, an integrative and functional medical expert, explains, "The body has an extremely difficult time breaking down casein." He further adds that "The common symptoms of dairy sensitivity due to casein are: excess mucus production, respiratory problems and digestive problems like constipation, gas, bloating, and/or diarrhea."[34]

Dr. T. Colin Campbell, coauthor of *The China Study*, goes a step further and says, "Through his studies he found casein to be the most relevant cancer promoter ever discovered."

4. Acne

"Acne is now an epidemic disease in Western countries, yet it is essentially nonexistent in populations who do not consume dairy products."[35]

Acne and allergies are most likely the cause of eating dairy products. They are more common in children who consume dairy products. Study after study has shown an association between dairy consumption and acne.[36]

5. Pus

Milk contains pus and antibiotics. "Cows are shot up with hormones and milked constantly, which regularly leads to infections in the udders. The result? Pus. Lots of it. One liter of milk often contains hundreds of millions of pus cells."[37] The pus is combated by using antibiotics, keeping the pus count below 750,000 cells per milliliter, an amount that is accepted by the United States Department of Agriculture (USDA).

The 2003 FDA Pasteurized Milk Ordinance (PMO) sets the maximum level of somatic cells allowed in Grade A milk at 750,000 cells per milliliter—a level that has been in effect since at least 1999.[38]

6. There are alternatives

"Perhaps the most compelling reason to avoid milk and dairy products is that they are completely unnecessary. Despite the incredible marketing powers of the Dairy Council, milk offers our bodies nothing that we can't get from natural plant-based sources."[39] Milk, yogurt, cheeses, and cream sauces made from almonds, soy, cashews, and peas can easily be made at home or bought from the grocery store.

In my experience, giving up milk and dairy products helped with my diverticulitis, chronic constipation, heartburn, reflux, and allergies.

C. Sugar

In his book *How Not To Die*, Dr. Michael Greger writes on page 328,

There are few popular diets out there that urge people to stop eating fruits because their natural sugars (fructose) are thought to gain weight. The truth is, only fructose from added sugars appears to be associated with declining liver function, high blood pressure, and weight gain. How could fructose in sugar be bad but the same fructose in fruit be harmless? Think about a sugar beet and a sugar cube. In nature, (sugar beet) fructose comes packaged with fiber, antioxidants, and phytonutrients that appear to nullify the effects of fructose.

Consuming sugar in fruit form is not only harmless, but actually helpful. Eating berries can blunt the insulin spike from high glycemic foods like white bread, for example. This may be because the fiber in the fruit has a gelling effect in your stomach and small intestine that slows the release of sugars or because of certain phytonutrients in fruit that appear to block the absorption of sugar through the gut wall and into your bloodstream. So eating fructose the way nature intended carries benefits rather than risks.

The isolation of sugar from the whole food may be the reason why you are more likely to supersize soda than sweet potatoes and why you are unlikely to eat too much corn on the cob, but can't seem to get enough high fructose corn syrup. The overconsumption of sugar sweetened fruits has often been compared to drug addiction.

Remember that old adage that "health is wealth"? That's really about leading a healthy, successful, and enriching life that is devoid of illness, anguish, and injury. I wish the same for you. So, I have blended experiences with evidence in an earnest endeavor to help you understand that egg, meat, dairy, and sugar are the biggest adversaries to one's good health, particularly when it comes to animal proteins.

I continue my argument as a votary of plant-based diet foods and the benefits it provides.

Nutrition and the Aging Process

Can we slow down the aging process so that we not only live longer but also healthier?

In order to answer this question, let's talk about aging. Each cell in the body has forty-six strands of DNA coiled into chromosomes. At the tip of each chromosome, there's a tiny cap called a telomere that protects our DNA from becoming ragged (damaged) or wearing out. From the time we are born, our cells divide; and each time they divide, a bit of the telomere is lost. Over time, they shorten until they are gone. And when the telomeres are gone, we die.

So, what can we do to protect and lengthen our telomeres? What can be done to prevent the telomeres from burning away too fast? The consumption of fruits, vegetables, and other antioxidant-rich foods has been associated with longer, protective telomeres. In contrast, the consumption of refined grains, soda, meats (including fish), and dairy have been linked to shortened telomeres.

The health of the telomeres depends upon the activity of the telomerase enzyme. Elizabeth H. Blackburn, PhD, who was awarded the 2009 Nobel Prize in Medicine for the discovery of telomerase, the enzyme that replenishes the telomere, found in a study partly funded by the United States Department of Defense, that three months of whole-food, plant-based nutrition and other healthy changes could significantly boost telomerase activity.[40] Also, weight loss through calorie restriction and vigorous exercise failed to improve telomere length. It was therefore determined that weight loss is due to the quality and not the quantity of the food eaten. *"In other words, it wasn't weight loss or the exercise that reversed cell aging, it was the food."*[41]

Athletes and Impact of a WFPB Diet

As an athlete, I was interested in what impact diet would have on athletes competing in extreme sports. The Roman gladiators had a diet that was mostly vegetarian, according to an analysis of bones from a cemetery where the arena fighters were buried. The study has been carried out by academics from the Medical University of Vienna in Austria and the University of Bern in Switzerland. The bones revealed that the typical food eaten by gladiators was wheat, barley, and beans—and this echoed the contemporary term for gladiators as the "barley" men.[42]

Humans are not genetically, anatomically, or physiologically adapted to eating meat-based products. We have longer digestive tracts than carnivores, and have trichromatic vision (ability to see three primary colors: red, green, and blue). The longer digestive tract helps us digest plant fiber, which requires longer processing time; and the trichromatic vision that enables us to see more colors assists us in finding fresh, ripe fruits and vegetables. Also, we cannot make our own vitamin C, which is only found in plant-based foods and fruits. In addition, we humans have teeth with the low cusps required for crushing and grinding plant tissues. Our teeth were not meant to eat meat like carnivores, which have teeth like scissor blades to shave off the meat.

To summarize, meats, dairy, and eggs are not required for optimal athletic performance. What is required is a diet high in carbohydrates, low in fat, and moderate amount of proteins.[43]

Soy Products and Estrogens

Patients often ask me about soy products and estrogen. In reality, soybeans naturally contain phytoestrogens called isoflavones.

Some people hear the word *estrogen* in the word *phytoestrogens* and assume that soy has estrogen-like effects. On the contrary, *studies show that a lifelong diet rich in soy foods reduces the risk of breast cancer in women. Soy contains protein, isoflavones and fiber, all of which provide health benefits.*[44]

WFPB Diet, Vitamin B12, and Vitamin D

I have a few thoughts about vitamin B12 and vitamin D for people on a WFPB or vegan diet. Plants do not make vitamin B12; bacteria in the soil, rivers, and streams make it. But because of industrialized farming and chlorination of water, we do not get B12 from the water or soil. The good thing is we do not get water-borne diseases either.

Regarding vitamin D, we can get all we need from the sun. Staying in the sun for about fifteen to twenty minutes each day is adequate to get your daily requirement. However, how many people are exposed to sun daily? *"In the United States, about 50 percent to 60 percent of nursing home residents and hospitalized patients had Vitamin D deficiency."*[45]

So it is advisable to take vitamin B12 and vitamin D in a supplement form, and it is prudent to get your vitamin B12 and vitamin D levels checked periodically.

Is Veganism a Fad?

In 2019, there were 600,000 vegans in the United Kingdom, or about 1.6 percent of the country's population. The US vegan population is growing at a rate of 600 percent.[46]

Around the world, consumers are becoming more aware of their health, the planet, and the animals, and search data from Google Trends show an impressive worldwide increase in the adoption of veganism. The leading vegan regions include the United States, the United Kingdom, Israel, Australia, Canada, Austria, and New Zealand.

This global shift to eating a plant-based diet has also attracted the attention of celebrities, such as Miley Cyrus, Joaquin Phoenix, Bill Clinton, Pamela Anderson, Stevie Wonder, Brad Pitt, Russell Simmons, Jennifer Lopez, Novak Djokovic, Bryan Adam, Mac Danzig, and the William sisters, Serena and Venus.

The 2018 report from the UK's Agriculture and Horticulture Development Board (AHDB) suggests the shift toward veganism and flexitarianism is being led by the younger generations. Record numbers of university students, for example, now follow a plant-based diet. However, as Food Navigator (a leading food publication) notes, there is research to suggest this is a long-term change and not just a passing fad.

A study by the Food Ethics Council in the United Kingdom revealed that 54 percent of young consumers believe the food system is fundamentally unfair to animals, as well as the environment and workers in developing nations. The council stated that food businesses will now have to change, not consumer attitudes.

As the executive director of the council, Dan Crossley said, "What we are seeing though is younger generations increasingly demanding food systems based on different values and participating in the food system in new ways. There is a moral imperative for food businesses to step up and ensure they are not treating others unfairly, whether that be people, the animals, or the planet."[47]

This perspective goes beyond the United Kingdom. In 2018, results compiled by leading retail data company Nielsen for the Plants Based Foods Association showed that US sales of plant-based food had increased by more than 20 percent over the previous year, topping US$3.3 billion. Also, plant-based dairy alternatives are an explosive-growing category, with 50 percent growth. This category includes plant-based cheeses, creamers, butter, yogurts, and ice creams, but not plant-based milk). Plant-based milk now represents 15 percent of the total milk market.[48]

Aside from eating habits, a widely cited 2013 report by the Food and Agriculture Organization (FAO) of the United Nations estimates about 14.5 percent of the annual global greenhouse gas emissions can be attributed to livestock. This is roughly equivalent to the emissions from all the fuel burned by the world's transport vehicles, causing a catastrophic effect on our environment.

> *Veganism has been around for thousands of years but it's not until the 1940's that the word vegan emerged to describe people who abstained from any form of animal cruelty.*
>
> *Greek philosopher Pythagoras was a huge advocate of plant-based living and this quote dates back to 500 BC: "As long as Man continues to be the ruthless destroyer of lower living beings, he will never know health or peace. For as long as men massacre animals, they will kill each other. Indeed, he who sows the seed of murder and pain cannot reap joy and love."*
>
> *Plant-based diets are environmentally sustainable, health promoting, and in perfect alignment with most peoples' moral codes. The vegan diet is certainly not a fad. It is definitely here to stay.[49]*

I would like to conclude this chapter with some specific comments and experiences from my own life with respect to eating a plant-based diet.

Being of South Asian descent, learning when I was fifty-six that I had heart disease made me take a second look at my life. Up until then, I had lived a couch-potato lifestyle, which comprised shunning any kind of exercise and gorging regularly on a carnivore diet (an all-meat diet). This had a disastrous effect on my body. However, since I turned around my life with the aid of regular exercise and the pursuit of a WFPB diet, my total cholesterol is 152, my high-density lipoproteins (HDL) has shot up from 29 to 57, and my blood pressure and triglycerides are normal.

In my seventy-three years, I have been admitted four times to the hospital. Once for open-heart surgery, twice for a perforated colon due to severe diverticulitis (inflammation of abnormal pouches in the large intestine), and once for acute urinary retention because of an enlarged prostate.

On my second perforation, I was advised by the surgeon to have part of my colon removed to prevent further attacks, even as I would have had to wear a colostomy bag for a few months. At the time, I was on intravenous antibiotics, my fever had come down, and I was stable. But after long discussions with my colleagues, I decided not to have the surgery. Instead, I decided to follow a plant-based diet. Since then, I have not had any medical problems. *Such are the miracles of a WFPB diet.*

In 2015, Dr. Kim A. Williams, the then president of the American College of Cardiology, was asked why he chose to eat a strictly plant-based diet. He said, "I don't mind dying. I just don't want it to be my fault."[50] Dr. Williams is one of the world's most famous vegan cardiologists who is an advocate of plant-based nutrition.

You can accept a plant-based lifestyle at any age, and you will reap immense benefits from that diet. I did it in my late sixties, and while I have never felt better, I wish I had adopted it earlier.

While growing consumerism and materialism, and increasing dependence on technology, is good economics, it has also had a negative impact on a personal level for many of us, leading to enhanced stress and anxiety.

The biggest protection against rising stress levels and surging heart disease cases is the adoption of a WFPB diet and regular exercise. By all means, follow what medical science or your physician prescribes, but there is no harm in experimenting with a plant-based diet for your inner well-being. After all, if doctors have all the answers, why have so many of them undergone an angioplasty or bypass surgery? Why do so many doctors suffer from high blood pressure?

Remember, no other diet has proven to reverse heart disease, our number one killer, as effectively as the WFPB diet. It therefore makes sense to switch to plant-based foods as the default diet for our kids and ourselves. It is important to get your kids to eat healthy. Start early, start young. Alternatively, make small changes in your diet. Small dietary changes will improve your health, keep you energized, and make you feel incredible. Try plant-based food today. I assure you it's tasty, and will also cut your grocery bill in half.

I would like to leave you with an important thought that will help you understand how probiotics *adversely* affect the gut microbiomes, that is, the microbes in our intestines.

Probiotics and Gut microbiomes

The gut microbiome weighs as much as five pounds, more than the human brain, and surprisingly, may have as much influence over our bodies.

There are trillions of microbes in our gut that coexist with us in ways that are still mysterious to us. They not only help process our food, but also help in making the vitamins, essential amino acids, and other nutrients our bodies require. In addition, they protect us from other bacteria, and in some intricate way they regulate our immune system. Their capacity to process the food we eat is linked to our health as well as our diseased states. Research suggests that a healthy microbiome may reduce our risk to diseases like diabetes and cancer.[51]

Doctors are already treating diseases by manipulating gut bacteria. One such example is the life-threatening infection or inflammation of the colon caused by clostridium difficile (C. difficile). This can be remedied by moving bacteria from the gut of a healthy donor to a sick person. Basically, a stool transplant.

Dr. Jeff Gordon at Washington University in St. Louis is recognized as "The father of the microbiome." During an interview with Dr. Jon LaPook that was featured on *60 Minutes* on Sunday, June 28, 2020, we learned that in a landmark experiment, Dr. Gordon and his team made a lean mouse fatter by giving it the bacteria of a fat mouse.

The CBS news program went on to say that "Millions of people are trying to improve their microbiomes themselves using probiotics, so-called good bacteria. *But here's the problem: there's a lot of conflict among scientists about whether probiotics provide any benefit at all.*" The health and science portion of the *60 Minutes* program further stated, "Probiotics is a $50 billion global industry sold to us in capsules, popsicles, cereal, tea and some yogurt. And we're told probiotics can even help your dog."

It takes guts to say that probiotics do not work in your gut. Dr. Patricia Hibberd, an infectious disease specialist and a professor of medicine at Boston University, emphatically stated in the same show that probiotics are not beneficial in reducing diarrhea from antibiotics, treating Irritable bowel syndrome (IBS), or in decreasing allergies. She added, "The whole idea that maybe throwing in good bacteria that we would take by mouth that hopefully would land in the right places in the GI tract and work with the immune system. We just don't know how to do any of that."

Also during the course of the interview on *60 Minutes*, professors Eran Elinav and Eran Segal of Israel's Weizmann Institute of Science stated that in their extensive research with control studies, where half the volunteers were given probiotics and half of them a placebo, they found that "The probiotics, as they go in, they just go out and they don't populate the gut."

So, I'm thinking, all you're getting is expensive poop, $50 billion worth.

Elinav and Segal also found that "Probiotics actually delayed the restoration of the bacteria of those individuals to what they had before as compared to individuals who took antibiotics and then did nothing."

The CBS show noted that "Probiotics are added to some baby foods and even infant formula." Dr. Frank Greer, professor emeritus of pediatrics at University of Wisconsin, stated in the interview, "We don't really know how probiotics work." When asked the question, "Is there any convincing evidence that adding probiotics to infant formula is good for the baby?", Dr. Greer replied, "My answer to that would be no."

So why are probiotics put in so many different products?

As reported on *60 Minutes*, "The Food and Drug Administration, the FDA, does not classify probiotic capsules as drugs. That means they do not have to be proven safe and effective."

We also learned from the show that last year (2019), Dr. Jeff Gordon's team reported that a special supplemental mixture of nutrients containing chickpeas, soy, bananas, and peanuts can repair the damaged microbiome of malnourished infants.

Before and after my heart surgery, I too had lots of gut problems, like chronic constipation, irritable bowel, acid reflux, and the infamous diverticulitis, which led to the two perforations and hospital admissions. Maybe because of my largely carnivorous diet, my gut microbiomes were damaged. But now with my avid following of a WFPB diet, there is a possibility I have repaired my microbiome, as I am free from all the above.

I end this chapter by reiterating its most important points

- Diet is more important than exercise.
- *Eating an unhealthy vegetarian diet is just as bad as consuming the flesh of any animal (red meat, poultry, and seafood).*
- Egg, meat, dairy, and sugar are the four biggest adversaries of your health.
- It is not bad genes that run in the family, it is bad diet that runs in the family. Even if you do have a high genetic risk, a healthy plant-based diet is capable of negating most, if not all, of the risk.
- The best diet to prevent and treat (or reverse) heart disease is a whole-food, plant-based diet.
- We are living longer but not necessarily living healthier. Transition to a WFPB diet to live longer and healthier.
- Follow a whole-food, plant-based diet and cut your grocery bill in half.
- Try plant-based food today. It isn't just healthy, it's filling and delicious too.

Addendum

This diet and nutrition chapter, chapter 7, may imply to some that I am talking about parts of the larger story, what can be called *wholeness.* I would like to stress not to focus on specific parts, like lowering your saturated fats, cholesterol, or blood sugar, as separate entities. The point of wholeness is that all the nutrients (macro and micro) in the food you eat are consumed together, which takes care of all the chronic manmade lifestyle diseases.

8

EPILOGUE

There is no growth without change, no change without fear or loss and no loss without pain.

—RICK WARREN

I HOPE THIS BOOK has given you, my readers, an opportunity to evaluate your lifestyle in terms of health. Throughout your reading of the book, we have journeyed together, and I believe you can now see the mistakes I made and are aware of a new path to a more fulfilled life.

In 2009, when I was sixty-one, my world came crumbling down. I had become a *victim of my own creation* after nearly two decades of unmitigated pursuit of pleasure and material possessions. I had become a patient of heart disease. This personal crisis forced me to make life-transforming changes at physical, mental, and spiritual level that could not have been prompted by ordinary circumstances. In 2010, this health and personal crisis helped me to revive, and by 2020 it enabled me to thrive. Through the latter part of the decade, I learned to become the *creator of my own healthy destiny,* a proponent of plant-based diets, positivity, and physical fitness to live a longer, healthier, and happier life.

Change is painful, and transforming from someone with an inflated ego into a person seeking equanimity was initially agonizing but now is pure joy. Reengineering the lazy slob I was into a marathoning, mountaineering, triathloning, and century-cycling athlete was at first intimidating but now is highly gratifying. Redesigning a materialistic life into a purposeful one that includes cooking and gardening (hobbies discovered during the COVID-19 isolation) was at the start challenging, but now provides fulfillment and happiness.

Before the reader is daunted by what may seem an insurmountable task toward achieving dietary or exercise *nirvana,* it's important to realize that most radical changes in life start with small steps. As Confucius, the renowned Chinese philosopher, stated, "The man who moves a mountain begins by carrying small stones." Most large changes become easier when they are undertaken a bit at a time (unless you are an extremely determined person). Small, repetitive changes are similar to small monetary investments that accumulate high returns over a period of time.

To be frank, I'm not expecting every reader of this book to follow my lifestyle. The path to my achievements is not a road map for others to follow. In this book, I endeavor to highlight the importance of physical and mental exercising while having fun at the same time. In many cases, beginning a new venture is the hardest part, but it becomes easier. Changing one's food habits as a part of healthy living is, in my opinion, even more daunting than starting an exercise routine. Here as well, beginning with small changes can be helpful.

I should emphasize that, like recovering from an addiction, changing to a different or a modified lifestyle will not always be a seamless undertaking. There will be times when you will succumb to the temptation of your old life and habits. However, as you reapply yourself to your healthy lifestyle routine, things that felt terribly important in the past will soon seem trivial.

I have found that lasting happiness does not come from unlimited possessions, or from how important or famous you are in a community or society. It comes from an active body, healthy eating, a positive mindset, a compassionate heart, a passionate curiosity for lifelong learning, the ability to step out of your comfort zone and face your fears, balance between materialism and spirituality, the capacity to look for humor in a time of crisis, the pursuit of meaningful goals, and more importantly, being supportive of the dreams, aspirations, and unconventional choices of your loved ones.

It is then that you escape the trap of a mundane existence, seek new adventures for a life of meaning and purpose, and enable Mother Nature to do surgery on you (rather than a physician) to create an *Open Heart*.

Live by my credo: *Adventure may hurt you, but monotony will kill you.*

ACKNOWLEDGMENTS

To my late parents, Salma M. Taherbhai and Mohamed M. Taherbhai, I am deeply indebted for the sacrifices you made to ensure that my siblings and I got the best education possible (even though you had no formal education), and that played a vital role in advancing my career and shaping my destiny. Your collective strength and resilience made you stand out from others, and your blessings have helped me overcome life's unexpected challenges.

To my lovely wife of forty-eight years and chief ally, Nafisa, I have no words to express my gratitude to you. Your ardent support held me together during the toughest adventures of my life. You have been there every step of the way, and I treasure our cherished association. I couldn't be more proud to be your best friend and husband. Thank you for bringing me down to earth each time my head was up in the clouds.

A big thank you to my eight-year-old grandson Kai Gehi, who ensures I stay young, vibrant, and energetic so that I have the stamina and strength to keep up with him, and have fun too.

I am grateful to my daughter, Anushka, and son, Nick, who have loved me unconditionally and supported me in all the physically daunting activities and adventures. They have participated in several activities. Nick and his friends joined me in the mud run and skydiving, while Anushka traveled to India to run alongside me in the Mumbai Marathon. I am blessed to have you both in my life.

A humble thank you to my brother, Husein Taherbhai, an author himself with several books to his credit. Your rewrites, constructive comments, and continual encouragement helped me believe in myself and bolstered my commitment toward writing this book.

To Fatima Mandviwala, my sister who departed this life in 2012 just before the Mount Kilimanjaro climb, I am eternally grateful for your unwavering support through the years. I know that you are forever watching over and guiding me with your loving spirit.

My appreciation to my nephews Mishal Pardiwala and Mikail Pardiwala, founders of TreeWear, a company that makes eco-friendly products that are beneficial for people and the planet. You introduced me to Instagram when TreeWear did an interview with me on heart-healthy lifestyle.

To my niece, Urvashi Punvani, who completed the Mumbai marathon with bleeding feet, demonstrating to the world that anything is possible if you put your heart to it. Thank you, my dear, for introducing me to a new dimension of determination.

Thank you to my nephews Nabeel Chatri and Munir Taherbhai and the team of Mona Shums, Jennifer Donald, and Sanjay Patel, who joined me and cheered me on at the Lake Lanier Triathlon in Atlanta.

A big heartfelt thank you, Dr. Bankim Patel, for journeying with me to Mount Kailash, Mount Kilimanjaro, and Pikes Peak. Your comforting words and sagacious advice during those arduous excursions helped me stay focused and successfully complete the climbs.

A special nod of gratitude goes to Vaishali, the leader of the Mount Kailash pilgrimage. You, Vaishali, have a small stature but are a power machine. Throughout the Mount Kailash journey, you encouraged us to soldier on with hope, faith, and optimism.

My deepest appreciation and thanks to my personal trainer, Stacey Garmon. *You are the best trainer anyone can have.* You saw something in me that I didn't. You guided me to improve my strength, endurance, balance, and flexibility. I am grateful to you for participating with me in the 5K, 10K, and half marathons, and the 100-kilometer and 100-mile bike rides.

Additionally, thanks to my friend and avid biker Naresh Purohit and my nephew Munir Taherbhai. You introduced me to clipless pedals and biking shoes when I first got on a road bike, and helped me learn to fall without getting hurt. Naresh, thank you for joining me on the 100-kilometer bike ride.

I am grateful to Dr. Pranav Mishra for training and for participating with me in the Nashville half marathon and the Chicago marathon.

I am also grateful to Dr. Ramesh Chellamuthu, a vegan who introduced me to intermittent fasting. He eats one meal a day and still has enough energy to play tennis most days of the week.

To the amazing David Ellis, thank you! To many, you are a small-town physical therapist, but to me, you are the best physical therapist in the world. Five weeks prior to the Boston marathon, I tore a calf muscle, which meant I could not run the marathon. Your zealous work and dedication were instrumental in getting me to the point where participation in the marathon became a real possibility, and then a reality.

I owe Dr. Diereck Sparks, an orthopedic surgeon in Gadsden, Alabama, a greater debt than I can express. You helped me with my running injuries without ever discouraging my newfound love for outdoor adventure.

A very special thanks to my office staff at Doctors Med Care of Gadsden, who after each adventure, made me feel like a "Million Dollar Man."

My sincere thanks to my patients. I am constantly learning and being inspired by you. Your remarkable capacity for resilience, tolerance, compassion, and empathy under adversity amazes me.

Thank you in abundance, The Art of Living Foundation, for teaching me pranayama, yoga, and meditation.

I owe a deep gratitude to the seasoned guides, porters, cooks, and the trekking group for their assistance, bonhomie, and commitment during our climbs of Mount Kailash and Mount Kilimanjaro.

I owe an enormous debt of gratitude to Shobha Swamy, a certified plant-based nutrition educator and consultant and an exceptionally good cook. You opened my eyes to the many delicious possibilities of a whole-food, plant-based, no-oil diet that can be as tantalizing to the taste buds as the foods I'd eaten for decades, and far more nutritious. Thank you also for helping fix my messy slides into an organized presentation for my interactive heart-healthy Zoom sessions.

To Naresh Wadhwani, I thank you for introducing me to the book *Dr. Dean Ornish's Program for Reversing Heart Disease* in 2006, when I was totally unaware that heart disease could be reversed.

A humble thank you to Uma Vullaganti and Dr. Alan Pernick. You believed in me from day one, and after hearing my story a few times, you were the first to suggest that I put my thoughts on paper. I am grateful to you for your timely reminders that led to the birth of this book.

A big heartfelt thanks to Lakshmi Devi Jagad, an able writer in her own right. Thank you for reading every word, those kept and those discarded—some several times over. You deserve the credit for giving me the idea of dedicating my book to my old self, Akil.

Special thanks to Pushpendra Mehta, for his valuable editorial and content insights. Thank you for your professionalism, enthusiasm, and patience as I navigated the unfamiliar world of publishing.

ABOUT THE AUTHOR

Akil Taher, MD, is a practicing physician in Gadsden, Alabama. He was raised in Mumbai, India, and trained in family medicine at the Flower Hospital in Sylvania, Ohio.

Dr. Taher is an eternal optimist, explorer, and adventurer, who in 2010, at the age of sixty-one, dramatically altered the conventional script adopted by most bypass surgery patients by undertaking a mountaineering trek to Mount Kailash in Tibet. This was a year after his open-heart surgery. In October 2011, he ran his first full marathon, the Chicago Marathon; and in September 2012, he climbed Mount Kilimanjaro, the highest free-standing mountain in the world.

Dr. Taher then expanded the canvas of his age-defying adventures by pursuing physically challenging activities on land, sea, and air, including a century bike ride (a 100-mile cycling event), triathlon, scuba diving, white water rafting, hang gliding, and skydiving. Over the last decade, he has overcome acute and chronic medical ailments by transforming his mind, body, and spirit through the adoption of a plant-based diet, practice of yoga and meditation, regular exercise, and developing a positive and purpose-driven mindset.

Dr. Taher is also a speaker focused on spreading the message of a heart-healthy lifestyle. *Open Heart* is his first book, and it chronicles his exploits since his heart surgery. He is happily married and has two children and an adorable grandson.

www.akiltaher.com   akil.taher48@gmail.com

NOTES

Open Heart *was written over a span of two years. In the course of my research, I read many books and articles. Should you see or observe any errors in the attributed quotes, references, or citations, please contact me at akil. taher48@gmail.com and I will be happy to correct the record.*

Endnotes

1 Emily Abbate and eds., "The Marathon Training Basics You Need to Know Before Your First 26.2-Mile, Race," *Runner's World*, February 12, 2020, https://www.runnersworld.com/training/a19599563/marathon-training-basics/.

2 https://www.ultimatekilimanjaro.com/blog/will-mount-kilimanjaro-erupt-again/.

3 Caldwell B. Esselstyn Jr. MD, *Prevent and Reverse Heart Disease: The Revolutionary, Scientifically Proven, Nutrition-Based Cure* (New York: Avery, 2008).

4 Tracie White, "Stents, Bypass Surgery Show No Benefit in Heart Disease Mortality Rates among Stable Patients," *Stanford Medicine News Center*, November 16, 2019, http://med.stanford.edu/news/all-news/2019/11/invasive-heart-treatments-not-always-needed.html.

5 Esselstyn, *Prevent and Reverse Heart Disease*, 102.

6 Craig M. Hales, MD, Margaret D. Carroll, MSPH, Cheryl D. Fryar, MSPH, and Cynthia L. Ogden, PhD, "Prevalence of Obesity and Severe Obesity Among Adults: United States, 2017–2018," *NCHS Data Brief*, No. 360, February 2020, https://www.cdc.gov/nchs/data/databriefs/db360-h.pdf.

7 "Nearly 7 in 10 Americans Take Prescription Drugs, Mayo Clinic, Olmsted Medical Center Find," *Mayo Clinic News Network*, June 19, 2013, www.mayoclinic.org.

8 Michael Greger, MD, "The Five Most Important Dietary Tweaks," NutritionFacts.org, March 23, 2017.

9 Kate Thayer, "South Asians Make Up 60 Percent of Heart Disease Patients: Everyone Knows Somebody Who Has Had a Heart Attack," *Chicago Tribune*, November 26, 2019.

10 Anahad O'Connor, "Why Do South Asians Have Such High Rates of Heart Disease?" *New York Times,* February 12, 2019.

11 Alka M. Kanaya, Eric Vittinghoff, Feng Lin, Namratha R. Kandula, David Herrington, Kiang Liu, Michael Blaha, and Matthew J. Budoff, "Incidence and Progression of Coronary Artery Calcium in South Asians Compared With 4 Race/Ethnic Groups," *Journal of the American Heart Association* 8, no. 2 (January 22, 2019), https://doi/10.1161/JAHA.118.011053.

12 "Emphasizing Prevention, Developing Therapies, Complementing Approaches," *Mens Sana Monographs,* 2005-2006, www.msmonographs.org.

13 A. G. Shaper and K. W. Jones, "Serum-cholesterol, Diet, and Coronary Heart-Disease in Africans and Asians in Uganda: 1959," *International Journal of Epidemiology* 41, no. 5 (October 2012): 1221-5.

14 T. Colin Campbell, PhD, and Thomas M. Campbell II, MD, *The China Study: Revised and Expanded Edition: The Most Comprehensive Study of Nutrition Ever Conducted and the Startling Implications for Diet, Weight Loss, and Long-Term Health,* (Dallas: BenBella Books, 2016), 79.

15 Esselstyn, *Prevent and Reverse Heart Disease*, 7.

16 Andrew Goddard, "Curative v. Preventative," *Medical Technology, News & Insights,* December 31, 2014, https://www.goddardtech.com/news-insights/curative-v-preventative/.

17 Kelly M. Adams, Karen C. Lindell, Martin Kohlmeier, and Steven H. Zeisel, "Status of Nutrition Education in Medical Schools," *The American Journal of Clinical Nutrition* 83, no. 4 (April 2006): 941S–944S, https://doi.org/10.1093/ajcn/83.4.941S.

18 Ali A. Sovari, MD, Jeffrey N. Rottman, MD, Russell F. Kelly, MD, Abraham G. Kocheril, MD, Arnold S. Baas, MD, Francisco Talavera, PharmD, PhD, Ronald J. Oudiz, MD, Krishna Malineni, MD, and Peter A. McCullough, MD, "Sudden Cardiac Death," *Medscape*, April 28, 2014, https://emedicine.medscape.com/article/151907-overview#a6.

19 Michael Greger, MD, and Gene Stone, *How Not to Die: Discover the Foods Scientifically Proven to Prevent and Reverse Disease* (New York: Flatiron Books, 2015), 4.

20 Kris Gunnars, "Protein Intake—How Much Protein Should You Eat Per Day?", *Healthline*, July 5, 2018, https://www.healthline.com/nutrition/how-much-protein-per-day.

21 Sofia Pineda, MD, "7 Ways Animal Protein is Damaging Your

Health," December 31, 2016, www. forksoverknives.com/wellness/animalproteindangers/.

22 Chuck Carroll, James Loomis, MD, and Susan Levis, MS, RD, "The Protein Myth, The Exam Room Podcast," *Physicians Committee for Responsible Medicine*, June 27, 2018, www.pcrm.org.

23 Carroll, Loomis, MD, and Levis, MS, RD, "The Protein Myth."

24 Michael Greger, MD, "How the Egg Industry Tried to Bury the TMAO Risk," *NutritionFacts*, December 31, 2019, www.nutritionfacts.org.

25 Kim A. Williams Sr., MD, interview by Dr. Pineda Ochoa, August 25, 2015, https://www.meatyourfuture.com/2015/09/williams/.

26 Melonie Heron, PhD, "Deaths: Leading Causes for 2017," Division of Vital Statistics, National Vital Statistics Reports 68, no. 6 (June 24, 2019), www.cdc.gov/heartdisease/facts.htm.

27 Carroll, Loomis, MD, and Levis, MS, RD, "The Protein Myth."

28 Mary H. Ward, Amanda J. Cross, Christian C. Abnet, Rashmi Sinha, Rodney S. Markin, and Dennis D. Weisenburger, "Heme Iron From Meat and Risk of Adenocarcinoma of the Esophagus and Stomach," *European Journal of Cancer Prevention* 21, no. 2 (March 2012): 134-138, https://pubmed.ncbi.nlm.nih.gov/22044848/.

29 Michael Greger, MD, "Plant Protein Preferable," *NutritionFacts*, November 1, 2011, https://nutritionfacts.org/video/plant-protein-preferable/.

30 Andrew Olson, "10 Reasons to Get Your Milk From Nuts Instead of Cows," 2014, https://www.oneingredientchef.com/10-reasons-avoid-milk/.

31 J. M. Chan, M. J. Stampfer, J. Ma, P. H. Gann, J. M. Gaziano, and E. L. Giovannucci, "Dairy Products, Calcium, and Prostate Cancer Risk in the Physicians' Health Study," *The American Journal of Clinical Nutrition*, 74, no. 4 (October 1, 2001): 549–554, https://doi.org/10.1093/ajcn/74.4.549.

32 "10 Reasons to Get Your Milk From Nuts Instead of Cows."

33 Elizabeth Weise, "Sixty Percent of Adults Can't Digest Milk," *USA TODAY*, August 31, 2009.

34 Heather McClees, "Casein: The Disturbing Connection Between This Dairy Protein and Your Health," October 2020, http://www.onegreen-planet.org/natural-health/casein-dairy-protein-and-your-health/.

35 "10 Reasons to Get Your Milk From Nuts Instead of Cows."

36 Clement A. Adebamowo‧ Donna Spiegelman, F. William Danby, A. Lindsay Frazier, Walter C. Willett, and Michelle D. Holmes, "High

School Dietary Dairy Intake and Teenage Acne," *Journal of American Academy of Dermatology* 52, no. 2 (February 2005), https://pubmed.ncbi.nlm.nih.gov/15692464/.

37 "10 Reasons to Get Your Milk From Nuts Instead of Cows."

38 "Is There Pus in Milk?" ProCon.org, https://milk.procon.org/questions/is-there-pus-in-milk/.

39 "10 Reasons to Get Your Milk From Nuts Instead of Cows."

40 US Department of Defense, US Army Medical Research Acquisition Activity W81XWH-05-1-0375, Fort Detrick, Frederick, MD, USA.

41 Greger, *How Not To Die*, 9.

42 Sean Coughlan, "Gladiators Were 'Mostly Vegetarian,' *BBC News,* October 22, 2014, https://www.bbc.com/news/education-29723384

43 *The Game Changers,* a 2018 documentary film about the benefits of plant-based eating for athletes.

44 Katherine Zeratsky, RD, LD, "Will Eating Soy Increase My Risk of Breast Cancer?", Mayo Clinic, April 8, 2020, www.mayoclinic.org.

45 Omeed Sizar, Swapnil Khare, Amandeep Goyal, Pankaj Bansal, and Amy Givler, "Vitamin D Deficiency," National Center for Biotechnology, April 28, 2020, https://www.ncbi.nlm.nih.gov/books/NBK532266/.

46 Darko Jacimovic, "28 Delicious Vegan Statistics to Savour in 2020," March 27, 2020, https://dealsonhealth.net/blog/vegan-statistics/.

47 Charlotte Pointing, "Vegan and Flexitarian Diets Are 'Here To Stay,' says New Report," August 2018, https://www.livekindly.co/vegan-flexitarian-diets-here-to-stay.

48 Ana Hanzek, "Retail Sales Data 2018," December 1, 2019, www.plant-basedfoods.org.

49 Maria Evripidou, "Veganism: Here To Stay or Just Another Fad Diet?", https://naturallysweetdesserts.com/veganism-here-to-stay-or-just-another-fad-diet/.

50 Jason Kelly, "Heal Thyself," *The University of Chicago Magazine,* January-February 2015, https://mag.uchicago.edu/science-medicine/heal-thyself.

51 Jonathan Lapook, "Do Probiotics Actually Do Anything?" *60 Minutes,* CBS, June 28, 2020.

Printed in Great Britain
by Amazon

79858179R00079